A Currawong Somersault

HEATHER WALKER

Copyright © Heather Walker 2021

All rights reserved. Apart from any use permitted under the Copyright Amendment Act 2006, and subsequent amendments, no part of this book may be reproduced by any process, stored in a retrieval system or transmitted by any means or process whatsoever without prior written permission from the copyright owner.

All characters names in this book have been changed for privacy reasons. All dogs however, are true to name.

Illustrations and Cover Design by Heather Walker
Typeset in Adobe Caslon Pro by Rob Walker

 A catalogue record for this book is available from the National Library of Australia

ISBN 978 0 6453457 0 4

For Robyn,

A cherished friend whose courageous spirit and generous heart make all other struggles pale into insignificance.

Contents

CHAPTER 1	Winter 2019	1
CHAPTER 2	Country Life 1970s	21
CHAPTER 3	Moving On	35
CHAPTER 4	Current Day	49
CHAPTER 5	Young Love	57
CHAPTER 6	Spring 2019	63
CHAPTER 7	With Challenge Comes Strength	75
CHAPTER 8	Farewell	81
CHAPTER 9	Cultural Hub	91
CHAPTER 10	Homecoming	109
CHAPTER 11	Summer 2019	121
CHAPTER 12	Trusting Your Gut	129
CHAPTER 13	A Getaway October 2019	141
CHAPTER 14	A New Year 2020	157
CHAPTER 15	Breaking News – Fire Crisis	175
CHAPTER 16	Summer 2020	183
CHAPTER 17	COVID-19	199
CHAPTER 18	Autumn 2020	215
CHAPTER 19	Easter 2020	229
CHAPTER 20	Winter 2020	239
CHAPTER 21	A Song Bird	251
CHAPTER 22	Open Space	271
CHAPTER 23	Uncertain Times	281
CHAPTER 24	Business Not As Usual	285
CHAPTER 25	Virtual Escape Lockdown	293
CHAPTER 26	Take 2 – Partial Lockdown	297
CHAPTER 27	Stamina	303
CHAPTER 28	Stage 3 – Melbourne Lockdown	311
CHAPTER 29	Lockdown Birthday July 2020	321
CHAPTER 30	Numbers Say It All	335
CHAPTER 31	The Plan	341
CHAPTER 32	The Best Is Yet To Come	353
CHAPTER 33	Bring On Spring	365

Recipes

1.	Mother Muesli	6
2.	Winter Hot Pot Soup	10
3.	Sweet and Sour Pork	30
4.	Apple Sponge	31
5.	Coffee Ice cream	52
6.	Ginger Fluff Sponge Cake	90
7.	Chicken and Mushroom Pie	151
8.	Scalloped Potatoes	153
9.	Italian Celebration Cake 'Migliaccio Napoletano'	154
10.	Gingerbread	171
11.	Devilled Eggs	173
12.	Waldorf Salad	174
13.	Apple Strudel in Filo	222
14.	Shanghai Braised Pork Belly and Rice	224
15.	Danish Honey Cakes	235
16.	Anzac Biscuits	237
17.	Blueberry and Coconut Muffins	245
18.	Zucchini and Mustard Fritters	246
19.	Vocal Tea Remedy	262
20.	Red Capsicum and Lentil Soup	318
21.	Sour Cherry Slice and Ricotta Honey Cream	334
22.	Orecchiette with Broccoli	351
23.	Salmon Pappardelle with Red Onion and Dill	374

Author's Note

The initial concept to write about Melbourne and inner city living was the catalyst to explore the fundamentals that make it the *World's Most Livable City*. I started with the idea that each season would highlight all the things that Melbournians hold dear – the love of sport, coffee, culture, arts, nature and the great outdoors – personalising this with my own experiences.

Little did I realise that in focusing on where I live I would also learn what mattered most to me. The year became like no other, when COVID-19 changed all of our worlds. For me, that meant shutting my fitness business and managing life differently.

Being contained in lockdown provided the time and space to evaluate what really matters and also take a long hard look at myself, bringing into context how the people and relationships involved in my past helped create who I am today. My Nanna's wisdom, my mother's care in providing food, my choir mistress who brought singing alive, all of these memories started to weave around current life and reminded me of the differences in how we now live our lives.

Strangely however, there were still fundamental things that remained the same. Both past and present highlighted we all share a common need, regardless of age and circumstance. We all need kindness, care and someone to reach out to.

It wasn't my intention to focus on the pain which had taken over my life for so long, but as the story evolved I realised it couldn't be hidden, as it seemed to sit in each chapter without saying a word. Lockdown brought a unique opportunity to create change in a big way. My story now includes getting off opioids; something which challenged me to the core.

Life can throw anything at us and turn us upside down in a heartbeat. We all share struggle in some form. It's seen in grief, loss, loneliness, self-doubt, anxiety, confusion and physical limitation. For me, pain highlighted many of these things and I can now understand that being honest with myself and working through difficulty has given me something unique. There's a healing that happens when you're willing to face your fears and this acceptance of self gives way to a humble gratitude. It highlights that even the smallest of things – a kindness, a smile, a bird's somersault – can give something so special; you feel you have received the gift of life.

My hope, dear reader, is that my Melbourne shines brightly in the livable stakes, and that in some small way, my experiences touch something in you that may lead to change. If this happens, please know that there is nothing to fear. If you choose to explore becoming your best self, you will find a strength from within that you didn't realise was there. Trust your inner self and know that you can get through anything.

So in a strange way, I am eternally grateful for the lessons I am learning, and grateful to the *World's Most Livable City* for opening up my eyes to see that it holds so much more than I could ever have imagined.

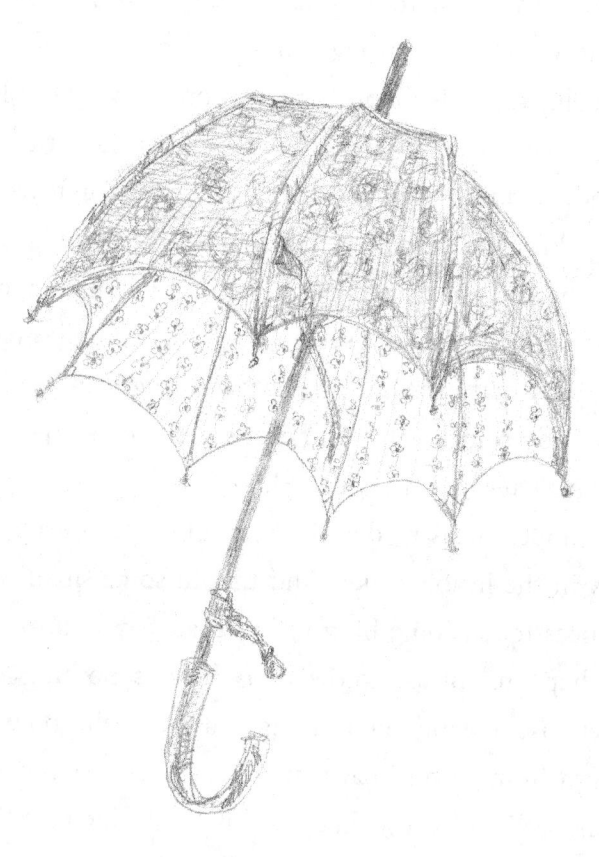

CHAPTER 1

Winter 2019

Melbourne's winter held its usual chill. The wind lashed at the flat tin roof and although I was snuggled up under the doona cover a shiver went through my body. Even the nearby cranes were not in operation, instead of digging deeper into the excavation below they hummed an eerie high-pitched song in the wind. The *World's Most Livable City* needed to hibernate. A momentary lull to progress. Five more minutes. A cup of tea was calling me to rise and Steve had very kindly placed a now very cold cup next to the bed a few hours before. There was no recollection of him doing this, so I sighed as I realised at last there had been a few hours of good sleep. Lately it seemed to be a constant catch up, elusive, uncomfortable and so unpredictable. I shared my life with chronic back pain, an unwelcome visitor who had moved in to stay after an unfortunate fall some years back. It's strange how everything seems to stay the same until it changes. We imagine that things will stay forever as they are, yet in a blink of an eye our world can be turned upside down. That's what happened to me. Wrong time, wrong place and a fall that left me suffering debilitating back pain. Steve and I were now both living around the demands that coping with pain required, restriction, disconnect and an ever-shrinking platform called life.

Two more minutes. Who was I kidding? I just didn't want to get out of bed, so pulled the covers over my head to muffle the rain pelting at the window. Grief, how could anyone be outside in this weather?

A distant train went through the nearby station and dinging bells signalled that the gates were down. Straight through it went. You've got to admire train drivers doing the hard yards rain or shine, they're probably up in the early hours. There's a lot to be grateful for. *Ok stop talking to yourself and get up.*

The covers flew back in one swoop. Less exuberant was the disembark process. First roll to the right, legs to the side and then over the edge, use your arms and then onto the feet. Done. Slide on slippers. Done. Cardigan, no maybe another top first and then cardigan. Ok good start. Tea.

WINTER 2019

The kettle boiled. English Breakfast is measured in the silver thistle spoon which belonged to my grandmother. Just a third is dispensed in the favourite white teapot and timed it's ready by the amount of time it takes to get the cup, find the saucer and retrieve the milk. We're nearly there. The white porcelain welcomes the pouring tea and settles so easily in the gold leaf saucer that for a moment I look at the wonder of it all.

Smell it … watch how the milk swirls into the tea, converging, enveloping and becoming the colour of choice. Therapy? … yes indeed it is. The thought that I've just morphed into my mother is pushed vehemently to the side with the first long refreshing sip.

Leaning against the kitchen bench, I survey the room with cup in hand. Steve's scarf is hanging over the chair, so he'll freeze on his return tram trip home later tonight. The blinds are all up at different heights in the lounge room below and already the windows and glass doors are glistening with the last burst of rain. This year seems to bear a fierce winter wind. Those blinds are going to have to be straightened up before anything else happens. Now breakfast.

Muesli is now the breakfast staple in our household, and although I would certainly prefer just a plain piece of sour-dough and vegemite with the morning cuppa – it's further confirmation I am definitely becoming my mother.

After spending a fortune on buying packaged muesli I discovered a way to reduce the cost and mix up the formula. It's simple. Buy two packets of organic oats and put three-quarters in a large sealed jar then add cinnamon, currants, dried coconut, chopped raw almonds, psyllium husk, chopped dried apple, pumpkin seeds and dried cranberries.

Mix it up and then use this as the Mother Muesli, topping up every few days with more oats. Delicious with yoghurt and milk.

This was a cunning plan to slow Steve's eating pace. After many years of marriage our family upbringings have only become more exaggerated as we've aged. He originates from a family of wild talkers who eat around their ever-increased conversation levels to the point where no one knows what's being said or what's being eaten. It's a flurry, a theatre, and if you're not up to pace his mother would whisk away a half finished plate mid-sentence.

In complete contrast, my family quietly pecked away at their meal giving each item on the plate the dignified respect each thing deserved, especially when so many less fortunate than us were going hungry. Conversation was considered, sparse and each person listened until all was said, even the ticking of the mantle clock sometimes waited patiently for a reply.

Consequently, as you have probably already imagined, there have been some interesting adjustments as our two worlds converged, especially around meals. Not always a success but often confounding or at best, amusing.

One such occasion was a Christmas celebration where all of Steve's family had congregated at the home of his sister Marilyn. Marilyn and Peter had just moved to a new home which had a postal business included in the deal and we all converged on the small country town to check it out.

Steve's parents, along with his elder sister Catherine, her husband Bill and Sally our young niece, gathered together with uncles and aunties who had not been seen for some time. Before long, noise levels increased beyond the small community's threshold, waking up all the neighbourhood chickens and causing them to squawk and cluck in agreement.

A donkey wandered down the street to check out what was happening and before anyone could finish piling their plates with seconds, it had decided to start eating the front garden.

At the same time, regardless of the kerfuffle, Steve's mother felt *now* was the perfect time to deliver the Christmas gifts. Amid the confusion of eating, receiving a gift, checking out the wildlife and making sure Marilyn's dog Boris hadn't escaped to bite the donkey, a wonderful time was had by all. This left me slightly winded and baffled, excited and mystified. This was chaos at its best. This was now my family and I loved every crazy minute.

Mother Muesli

Ingredients:

2 packets organic oats (1 for reserve)

1 tablespoon ground cinnamon

1 tablespoon dried shredded coconut

1-2 tablespoons organic psyllium husk

1 tablespoon dried currants

1 tablespoon chopped raw almonds
½ tablespoon dried cranberries
½ tablespoon dried organic chopped apples
½ tablespoon pumpkin seeds

Method:

Fill a large glass jar (with a good seal) with oats to ¾ full.

Add half the above ingredients at a time and give a good shake, then add the rest and shake again, then simply top up with some more oats.

Top up the jar with raw oats every couple of days and shake through ingredients each time.

When the mix is starting to appear more oat based, just top up a few of the ingredients to your taste.

Serve:

Serve with organic yoghurt or probiotic yoghurt.

A little milk.

A few fresh chopped strawberries and blueberries, or ½ banana and a drizzle of honey

It's hard to believe it's been more than 10 years we've been living in our inner-city apartment. Melbourne has been home for many years now and we are very proud of the place and with over 4.8 million in residence we are the most populated state of Australia with 453 people per square kilometre.

Inner-city living has both rail and tram on our doorstep making easy access to the city centre only 10 minutes away. Even in the last five years there have been radical changes around our area, with cranes and apartments fighting for position, slowly and systematically chipping away at the skyline, making sunlight a prized possession. The fundamentals remain the same however, with cafés, restaurants, fashion and variety stores and the Prahran Market within walking distance at the end of our street.

It's wonderful to walk around the corner to a café, to enter and be just getting settled to check the morning news when the barista brings your coffee just the way you like it, even without having to order. Perfect.

There's a gorgeous little French café not far from us that adds a flourish of two tiny madeleines, either orange or pistachio. French speaking and so chic, the staff give the impression that you also might be just as French as they are. All of a sudden you find yourself somewhere else. The soft pink walls are striped with tiny roses between, giving the impression of delicate intricate clouds. And then there are the glass displays filled with chocolate éclairs, macarons of every flavour, tarts and baguettes. Sadly the illusion slips away as my own accent intrudes and echoes in the space, but nonetheless my head lifts a little higher and there's a sense that perhaps my denims now look slightly more stylish than on arrival.

Walking around this area is something I have perfected and there are a number of routes that must surely recognise me by now, and most of them incorporate gardens of note, interesting and varied architecture and of course a puppy dog or two. It doesn't matter which direction, the smaller streets that run off the main roads display Victorian weatherboard houses with verandas covered in wisteria, red-brick cottages with white iceberg roses and lavender, and modern concrete designs with glass reflections hitting every angle, accentuating their clean lines.

Picket fences reside next to high concrete slabs and then a wonderful white and blue fence appears in view. A house with a wonky handwritten sign advertising 'airspace for sale' that has only just replaced the 'house for sale' one that sat for months on show. It's intriguing how the Greek community take selling to a completely new level. Even the trunks of the lemon trees that line the front of the house either side are painted white to match the white fence line. The roof and window frames are a proud sky-blue. Nothing has been spared the white and blue theme and I often wonder whether the inside reflects the same?

Maybe the dining room table is blue and the chairs white? The concrete in the rear patio would have to be whitewashed, with grapevines trailing overhead.

Perhaps in another 30 years climate change may bring the sea to their doorstep to complete the dream home as the owners imagine it to be.

In the next block on the corner is a tumbledown house and matching wooden fence with trees that dangle over onto the pavement, bottlebrush that have been let go to do their own thing, untamed, wild and beautiful. A mysterious place that appears to hold many secrets. The only hint that there is life within presented itself by chance, when an old tin with bay leaf twigs was left at the front gate with a sign inviting anyone to please help themselves.

How fortunate and timely to be making stockpot soup which required a fresh bay leaf. Pot complete, thanks very much.

Winter Hot Pot Soup

Ingredients:

1 cup buckwheat kernels, rinsed clean
1 generous pinch dried chilli flakes
1-2 fresh or dried bay leaves
1 brown onion, coarsely chopped
1 clove garlic, chopped
2 waxy potatoes cubed
2 thick slices butternut pumpkin, cubed
2 large carrots cut into coins
1 medium head broccoli cut into florets and/or
2 zucchini cubed
10-12 green beans cut
½ cup frozen peas
4 cups boiling water or stock of choice
Parsley roughly chopped and thyme
(or other favourite herbs)

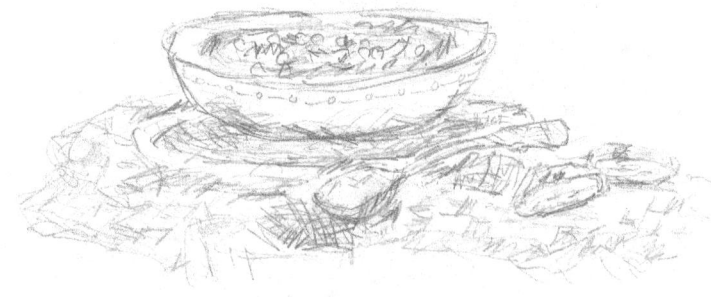

Method:

Wash and prep all veggies.

Heat a tablespoon extra virgin olive oil in a rather large saucepan.

Start by adding the onion, garlic and dried chilli flakes.

Cook until just fragrant and slightly soft.

Add the buckwheat and work it around so it's coated with the oil and onion garlic mix. It should smell nutty and may pop as it heats.

Check for medium heat. Then add potato and cook for a minute, moving it around. Then add the pumpkin.

(The denser the veggies the more time they need. Last are the greens as they won't take as long and need to retain a little crunch for goodness.)

Add boiling water and/or stock and bay leaves.

Allow to boil for a few minutes.

Skim any froth on top and then add some greens. Leave the beans, peas, parsley and any other herbs until about 5 minutes before serving to stay crunchy.

Simmer for 30-35 minutes until veggies are soft, skimming froth throughout. May need to add more water.

Serve:

Serve steaming hot with crusty bread or toast.

This makes a large amount so it's great to freeze when cold or good to share with others.

Another block and it's either a right or left turn. Left leads towards Chapel Street and another favourite café, or around more streets with houses, dangling red roses, veggie gardens with concrete white pedestals, apartment blocks with small terraces, cooking smells and the occasional grass allotment with a few straggly grasses or shrubs tucked in a corner.

Frankie, an eight-year-old white highland terrier, lives in a beautiful Victorian house just near the café. When luck and all the moons align she can be found lying panting in the sun either on the path inside the front gate or under a bush to the left of the rose garden. She loves nothing better than to lie on her back and have her tummy scratched, all the while her little tail quivering and moving to the best scratch vantage point.

Inner-city Living

One of the very quirky and strange things about living in our apartment is that for some reason the design, built over 25 years ago, neglected to consider that anyone living there may actually like to cook. Not only do we as a group of apartment dwellers share the 13 steps that lead to our entries, but we are also privy to all the cooking smells that escape each kitchen via their front doors.

The rigmarole unfolds. It's a good day to roast a leg of lamb, slightly chilly weather and a couple of rosemary twigs picked on my last walk were the inspiration. There are just enough potatoes, some pumpkin, onions, lemon and frozen peas to seal the deal, so all placed in a high oven with everything dressed to perfection. Thirty minutes.

Now commences my partner Steve's worst nightmare. He feels the cold. Even with jeans tucked into his ugg boots, woolly jumper and many other layers underneath that, there is the need for a rug to cover head to toe so he doesn't freeze alive.

It's now time to check on the cook up. Taking a deep breath it's a quick step to the front door to open and secure, then whiz down to the courtyard glass door and open that. Run six steps up to the kitchen, take glasses off, put light on and with gloves now on, open the oven door to a woof of hot smoking air and shut as quickly as possible. Wait two to three seconds.

Steve is now in overdrive and the rug is over his head as he has frozen solid – all except his voice. Working quickly now, it's open the oven again, take out the smoking leg of lamb, turn it over, move things around a bit and slam the door shut. Complete. It's very wise indeed to never wash clothes on a big cooking day. Well, that is unless you'd like to smell of something to eat. Before the open all doors cooking plan came into being there had been times when we could have eaten our pillow halfway through the night, it smelt so convincingly of lamb. It begs to ask why you'd install an exhaust fan that goes absolutely nowhere?

There are many things happen that don't make sense. The non-functioning fan was a simple mistake, but whether a cost saver or perhaps stupidity, it caused a roll-on effect for me, because cooking became a major exercise. Whether it's small or large, we could turn ourselves inside out if we focus too hard on *why* something is the way it is. When something happens to us that changes our world and asks us to adapt, we have choice. A shock, a crisis, an accident, an illness can stop us in our tracks. Why me? Why now? Stuff does happen, and often. The interesting thing is how we deal with a long-term challenge.

There's an initial adjustment made when something happens to us because in the moment that's all we can do. We deal with it. However it's the years that follow that create the biggest challenge. For me, the medical path was based on physical treatment and having to find alternative ways to move and manage even the simplest of daily activities. I never would have dreamed that going to the toilet could bring such dread. Sitting was a nightmare and this simple function brought me to a screaming halt.

It's in the everyday workings of life where dealing with pain affects me. There are constant adjustments as I negotiate how best to conserve energy to get the best out of my day. Apart from the long list of my mood changes that Steve could relate, there have been a couple of stand-outs that were unexpected.

Most need a very robust sense of humour to cope with them.

When pain levels surge or peak above the normal level of acceptance a wave of heat surges through my body at a rate that could bowl over or singe any birds flying around my perimeter.

Technically speaking, I'm being assisted by a *very* supportive, and over-efficient sympathetic nervous system that thinks it has to rush to my aid and deliver some kind of response.

It thinks … Hang on a minute, something's not right here, I'll just step in and make sure this human comes to no harm! Time and again it takes over, until it programs a response. My poor old parasympathetic system doesn't even get a look in, and that's the one that *should* be overseeing proceedings.

It's this heat that makes me instantly strip off, open any door or window nearby and suck in as much air as possible to regroup without passing out.

Not a pretty sight and very difficult for Steve to witness. It's times like these that there are no questions to be asked of me, nothing can be done and time and its passing is the only relief on offer. Thankfully, there are some unique distractions that can help ease some of the pain and many of them have four legs.

Many dogs live in our area and among them a variety of owners who complement the style of dog they own.

Some however buck that trend and prove that inner-city

living is a place for rebels, for those who challenge the norm.

We love, love, love dogs and have a wish list which incorporates a dog or dogs of small to medium size with wiry, woolly or shaggy hair that resembles or doesn't our previous dog Bitey, a highland terrier. This dog will be a female for me and a male for Steve but will be so very well behaved that it definitely *won't* be getting on the bed or couch and *will not* accept food treats that we are eating. As yet the idea is still being formulated and negotiated therefore no actual breed has been decided.

Fortunately the dogs in our apartment block do like to come into the kitchen to check out the smells at the opening of the oven door scenario. It's a quick exchange of greeting, mostly sniffing and jumping. There's mild embarrassment for the owner who hovers at the entry unsure whether to follow inside or coax their dog outside with treats. A dilemma, but charming nonetheless.

Louis has to be the favourite offender. He's a small, stocky, pug-style puppy, with a curly tail that unravels when he's excited. Absolutely adorable. His owner defies the idea that dogs and owners resemble each other as she is tall with the longest legs you've ever seen in the shortest shorts imaginable.

Blonde, vivacious and brown most months of the year, she has a wonderfully lopsided smile which infects you without even realising it. Along with this charming ability she also makes an incredible latte and works tirelessly at the corner café down the street. Louis' best mate is a dog by the name of Ned, and his owner is also a mismatch in the looks department.

Ned lives in a lower level apartment from ours. He is a large dog, brindle in colour with a long snout and long tail. He was rescued by his owner. I don't know from where but quite clearly he has found what he needed in his current home. When he arrived he was very scared and skitsy and barked out of fear, then slowly over time the transformation happened.

It's nothing to now see and hear Ned and Louis running at full pelt up and down the lower level carpark chasing each other for all they're worth. Get out of the way when this is happening or you'll get knocked over! It's worth seeing from behind the safety of your car though, as the sight of the little legs and tongue darting around the large athletic frame has us all in stitches.

Pure unbridled happiness, dog style. You'll hear Ned's owner yelling 'Ned, Ned, slow down Ned … look out … you'd better move out of the way or they'll bowl you over!' I do move away as she suggests, but I wouldn't miss the spectacle for anything. It's hilarious!

There's only one cat residing here that I'm aware of though it hasn't been sighted lately. It's black. Very sleek. Green eyes. Very aloof. Not knowing much about cats, it's hard to describe the workings of what may be a shared conversation. There have been a few stare-offs and hasty retreats with a quick look back before darting away into the unknown – and that was just the cat.

Strangely though, the cat has crossed our threshold three times, and yes, you are right to assume that once again the front door was open, and yes, there were probably cooking smells of some description. But Steve cried out the last time, when all of a sudden we realised that it had darted inside and taken ownership of the marble serving table, halfway between the dining and lounge rooms. Another stare-off ensued.

Perhaps more was conveyed in the last look? Who knows ... but like a flash it was out the door and scampering back down the walkway. Very curious indeed.

Black cats conjure up all manner of thoughts and in recollection, this is the third black cat I've met over the years.

The first was cross-legged on the floor at show-and-tell in primary school. One lucky young girl brought in her kitten to show off and emphasise the fact that not *everyone* was lucky enough to have a pet. I had focused hard on nothing else but willing the kitten to come and sit in my lap. This was no mean feat as the kitten had to climb over a number of other bodies to get there, but get there it did and settled down until the end of every child's presentation was given. Absolute bliss. Weirdly, I felt some kind of mystical power which was more special than owning the kitten itself.

It had chosen me. It snuggled into my lap. I could feel its warmth and purring. I felt special because of this and so very happy.

The second cat lived next door. Mrs Ubergang was old. Really old. And her cat was probably as old as she was as it didn't move all that fast and would often be found in our place curled up in the sun under the water tank stand.

It had favourite spots which were easy to find as she stayed there so long it flattened out the area. She didn't run away. She wasn't completely black but had one white paw. The right front one, which looked like a conductor orchestrating some complex symphony in her own head when she waved her paw about.

She could conduct a whole orchestra of flies on a hot windless day, swatting the paw from head to ear, from ear to nose and back again. All the while her body stayed still, conserving every bit of energy left, except an occasional twitch of her tail, like a flick, random and unexpected.

We had many meaningful conversations together about growing up and why things were the way they were.

You can learn a lot from cats.

They're smart and very good listeners. Perhaps it's just the black ones that possess this unique quality, but I often wondered about the tail. Even though I didn't say anything to puss, I wondered whether she was irritated with something?

Her green eyes didn't change, they just blinked lazily or closed.
There was no clear sign that the conversation was the issue.
It was a mystery and something I thought about a lot.

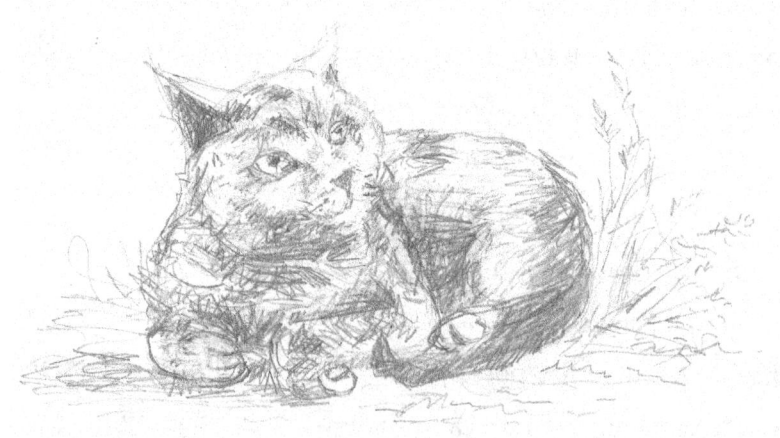

CHAPTER 2

Country Life 1970s

It's funny how animals can hold so much mystery for a child. It doesn't matter whether you live in the country or the city, animals give something to us that is not easily explained. There's a connection that happens when human and animal somehow understand each other. Animals interact and understand situations in a completely different way to us, but they can touch us deeply and bring about healing. Rebel, a dapple white horse, comes to mind, and he was huge or at least that's how it felt to me at the time.

A friend, Mandy Stevens, housed Rebel in her backyard. We'd sit high in a tree nearby singing songs of our own making, sipping our lemonade through soggy paper straws and hiccuping between verses. 'Someday I'm gonna write [fwit-boing], the story of my life [fwit-boing].' Laughing so hard we'd go limp and have to hang on so we didn't fall out and break our necks. On one occasion, after some persistent coaxing by Mandy, it was decided we'd try riding Rebel bareback down the lane next to where she lived.

It was quiet with no traffic. Up to this point my experience with animals was limited to a kitten sitting in my lap and a turtle and rabbit loaned by the school for one day. Standing next to Rebel's rump or almost under it brought reality to a screaming halt. How in the heck was anyone supposed to get on top of that! At this point running in the opposite direction as fast as possible seemed like a very good idea.

Easy for Mandy, she could ride, no problem. She angled the horse next to a gate and told me to get on that way. She was already on top. How did that happen? Rebel's tail mesmerised me and was flicking in my face. Then there were two bodies on the back and now the tail was flicking my legs causing them to itch like mad and there was no way anyone could scratch and let go at the same time. Now what?

What happened next was a blur that started with a slow walk and Rebel's rump moving around so much I was squeezing her to death from behind. Feeling confident, Mandy flicked the rope she'd tied around his neck and then we bounced around so aggressively that I had to close my eyes tight to stop my teeth chattering. This was not yet fun.

Then without warning we slipped. It was in slow motion. Sound seemed to warp into an underwater muffle, burbling and pounding in my ears causing tears to run uncontrollably. Our screams were somehow elongated, black and white, wafting out of our mouths, eyes blinking wide and then the world changed to technicolour topsy turvy. We were screaming with all our lungs now as we found ourselves upside down underneath the horse and I didn't like what I could see! Still clinging on like mad we hung there for what seemed like an eternity ... yelling 'stop, stop, stop', or 'wooh, wooh boy' in horse terms.

And then all of a sudden we were both on the ground. Rebel was towering overhead, hooves were going everywhere and then we banged our heads together, nearly passing out. After crawling out, checking all bruises and nursing the scratches I walked home slowly, thinking deeply about what had just happened to me.

As I entered the back veranda ready to explain to my mother a version of it all, I knew there was something to learn from this. I told her I had made a firm decision that from now on only animals lower than knee height would be my preference.

My mother dabbed the stinging cuts and bruises with Dettol, agreeing that probably would be wise. Very wise indeed.

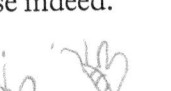

Country Living

The joy of country living in the seventies. Something that not every child gets to experience these days. Times have changed. Changed beyond recognition.

There were no helicopter parents. No information overload. No phones, and certainly not the carry-with-you variety. Yes there was television, going to the pictures or drive in, but these were seen as an occasional treat and not done all the time. Most of our time was spent outdoors, riding up and down the street on bikes, swimming in the nearby irrigation channel or playing in the piles of dirt waiting for roadworks to be done.

I could be seen dancing on the nature strip in old petticoats and hats making up songs and plays to entertain any passer-by. Play time was about making something out of nothing. Anything was possible with imagination and boredom was a word not used in our vocabulary. Idyllic as it all sounds, we also had responsibility.

There were jobs that had to be done and every child had certain things they had to do each week. The list was long and included cleaning up your room, sweeping, washing, dusting, collecting vegetables, mowing the lawn, washing the dishes, and even though there were sometimes quarrels, everything eventually got done. It had to, there was no real choice in the matter. Nothing to negotiate as kids were quite often seen but not often heard.

No one was remotely interested in what a kid had to say. We had to earn the right to be heard and we understood we had to respect our parents and elders as being the ones in charge.

Not always easy, but we knew our place and in some ways this took away the stress of decision-making. 'Be grateful for what you are given', 'Listen when you're being spoken to', 'Close your mouth when you're eating', 'Do your homework', 'Treat others the way you would like to be treated', 'Go to your room and think about what you have done', 'Eat your dinner or go without.'

The list goes on and on and many of these directives were non-negotiable. They seemed tough at the time and totally unreasonable, but somehow we all survived. Survived to cope with disappointment. Survived to deal with loss. Survived to understand that the world revolves around many other people than ourselves, and what we wanted. Survived to appreciate the time and effort our parents put into teaching us.

Survived without needing therapy.

Meal times were often a time of conflict and tension in our household because with two brothers who were older and wiser there was never an opportunity to win an argument, and there was no point even trying, as they knew the lay of the land and how to work the rules to their best advantage.

There was soon competition between siblings as to who could eat up their dinner the fastest so they could then enjoy dessert, if luck had provided any. There's no dessert if you don't eat all your dinner so there was no better incentive as treats were few and far between.

This was put to the test when dinner comprised brussel sprouts and cooked liver with onions. Even the smell was enough to make us gag, but eat it we did, chewing round and round our mouths in the effort to somehow get it down, purely because we knew there was roly poly jam tart to follow if we did and an extra dollop of cream if our plates were clean.

Our Nanna and Grandad lived a couple of streets away from us and Nanna was an amazing cook. We would always be on our best behaviour whenever we visited them for lunch, as her desserts comprised an entirely different repertoire. We would eat *anything* we were given in the hope of honey roll, fairy cakes, vanilla slice or the best of all, ginger fluff sponge.

Doing the dishes was an everyday chore for us and one which usually created some tension. Washing was the preference, as this took no time at all. No one wanted to dry because at this stage, all we wanted to do was get outside and play, therefore there was another trade-off, a system of bargaining or bartering. Something for something else.

Sometimes even pocket money was exchanged to get out of that one. But not often, as money, like dessert, was hard to come by.

Mrs Cook

My mother had a strong sense of commitment towards others. She helped many people in the small community, and as a young girl I learnt the importance of care in action. Talking about something was all well and good, but if it wasn't followed through, then it wasn't worth a great deal, as talk was cheap.

From an early age, I would help my mother carry the wicker basket full of food to a neighbour who wasn't well. The smells of lamb or pork casserole and veggies wafted in the air as we walked. This could be anywhere in the neighbourhood and walking the distance sometimes took a long time, making me feel very hungry by the time we had arrived to knock on the door.

I was always grateful to arrive and sit in a chair to rest. Perhaps there'd be a glass of water if I was lucky. There was nothing to do but observe. My mother would unpack the contents in a measured way, all the while chatting quietly to the lady we visited, looking around as she went, cleaning up the dishes that were on the bench and putting the kettle on for a cuppa. She'd brought milk and sugar just in case and some homemade biscuits. A quick inspection of the fridge showed it was almost empty. On this occasion it was Mrs Cook. She was a small round woman who couldn't move around a lot due to her hip. She used a stick but she seemed very wobbly on her feet.

My mother wrapped the crochet rug around Mrs Cook's lower body and proceeded to pour the tea and serve biscuits. I was hoping I would get a biscuit but, when nothing was given, spent my time looking around me instead.

I didn't know Mrs Cook and didn't understand much of the conversation, but I sat quietly looking at the lemon-coloured kitchen cupboards with worn wooden knobs, the tins of different sizes and colours stacked on the bench and the faded cream curtains that hung over the one window in the room. I wondered about Mrs Cook. Did she live alone? Where was her family? Did she have a cat?

On the way home I thought a lot about what I had seen but didn't know how to ask my mother about it all. I needn't have worried because she explained that Mrs Cook wasn't well and didn't have any family as her husband had died a few years ago.

She was like Mum and didn't drive, so she relied on walking everywhere, and this made it difficult to even get the bare essentials. She explained that when we got home, we would make a list and go into our garden and pick some of our veggies and fruit and take them to her the following day.

She thought it would be nice if I made a card or did a drawing for her to cheer her up, as she didn't have any children of her own.

This was one of many tasks that fell to me around the visitation routine. There were cards, drawings and sometimes

I would make up a poem or prepare a short song if the moment was right. Whatever the requirement, I felt needed and worked side by side with my mother to help those around less fortunate or in need of a pick me up.

Beef casserole, sweet and sour pork, chop suey or meat loaf featured heavily as they were meals in their own right and didn't need much to go with them, except a few beans or spinach from our veggie patch.

Sometimes there was a rhubarb and apple sponge, date loaf, or oat and spice biscuits depending on our finances at the time and what was available in the garden, but overall it felt special and was always gratefully received.

As I grew older, I was soon involved in the cooking and preparation of things. I didn't realise it at the time but these were lessons I would carry with me over many years.

The giving didn't just happen once or twice but continued as the need arose. It was a commitment of time. It was given in a spirit of respect. It was a bond of trust. I learnt that care related to giving of self and giving of time without any other reason than helping those in need.

Sweet and Sour Pork

Ingredients:

1 kg lean diced pork

1 brown onion sliced

¼ cup sugar

½ cup white vinegar

2 tablespoons soy sauce

1 small tin pineapple pieces drained

1 cup water

1 garlic clove diced

1 packet dried chicken noodle soup mix

Method:

In a pan fry pork in a little olive oil until browned.

Add onion and garlic until softened and fragrant.

Transfer the pork, onion and garlic to a medium size saucepan and add all other ingredients.

Simmer together for about 2 hours. Stir occasionally and add more water if needed.

Serve:

Serve with steamed jasmine rice or mashed potato.

Steamed beans.

Apple Sponge

Ingredients

3-4 large apples (either Granny Smith or mix with a sweet red variety)

1 tablespoon margarine or soft butter

½ cup caster sugar

1 egg

A little milk and pinch salt

1 cup self-raising flour

¼ teaspoon finely grated nutmeg

Method

Oven 190°C (170°C fan forced). Peel and cut apples into chunks.

Cook until firm in a medium size saucepan with 2 tablespoons of water for 2 minutes. Set aside.

Use a medium square or oblong dish and rub inside with margarine or soft butter.

In a medium size mixing bowl cream together sugar and margarine until light in colour and combined.

Add egg and beat well. Add pinch of salt and 1 tablespoon milk and beat again.

Sift self-raising flour and grated nutmeg into bowl and gently fold in. Don't overwork.

Place cooked apples into baking dish.

Check batter and add 2nd tablespoon milk. Gently mix. Texture should be 'easy pour'.

Cover the apple mixture with batter and bake 20-30 minutes until golden.

Serve with whipped cream or vanilla ice cream.

Even though cooking featured heavily in my upbringing it didn't fall easily into my list of skills. I would help my mother of course, and do what was expected of me at the school home economics class, but to my horror, by the time I was married and expected to provide something edible on the dinner table the list of workable recipes was very limited.

Tuna mornay and meat loaf were two dishes that my husband Steve somehow endured meal after meal.

True love can be measured in many ways but his acceptance of my inadequate skills was a testament to his vows for better for worse and thankfully the repertoire was never tested to the point of in sickness and in health.

To this day neither of us can bear the sight or smell of either of these dishes, and over time I embraced BBQ with salads and spent more time practising my mother's recipes.

There was often a frantic call to clarify what the heck had gone wrong with the custard or find out why the sponge hadn't risen as expected. Fish 'n' chips was a treat that my family rarely enjoyed so in the early days of marriage a strong relationship was forged with the local take-away to fill in the gaps.

Today is a very different day and the joy of cooking is now something that brings me pleasure, happiness and a sense of purpose, through sharing it with others.

COUNTRY LIFE 1970S

No matter where we live, food brings with it a wonderful connection and at times, the mixing bowls had just settled into their new environment when the process of packing up started all over again.

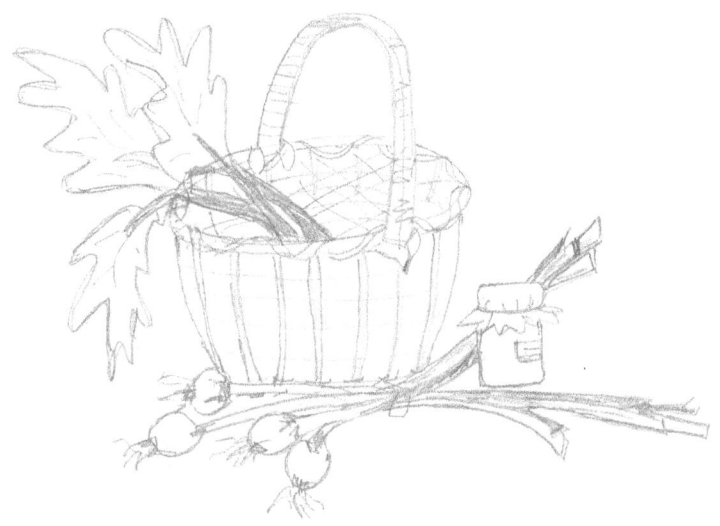

A CURRAWONG SOMERSAULT

CHAPTER 3

Moving On

What's a five-year plan anyway?

Moving from Adelaide to Melbourne was one of the best things that Steve and I decided to do. We'd outgrown what was then known as the Garden State, or perhaps the gardens had overtaken us with a sleepiness that had brought life to a standstill. The 1990 recession we had to have definitely had an impact, as we had to sell our home as a result of this.

Either way, it was change that was needed and a couple of new jobs presented that opportunity. Moving was in Steve's DNA and so this was just another one to add to the list. It was a studio management job for Steve and the well-known professional a cappella singing group Vocamotion, for myself. Bitey Boy, our white terrier, would soon clock up house number seven with this move, but as we already knew, this eight-year-old puppy was very adaptable. A little moody, very unpredictable, absolutely adorable, handsome, charming when food was on offer, wildly feisty and very, very adaptable. Whoever it was that discovered the parallels between matching dog and dog owner certainly uncovered a major truth in our household.

I had married my dog.

This became obvious at meal times in particular. First the smells would bring in one body, and then the other followed not long after. Two of a kind. Fortunately however, the little black lips and wet black nose were only apparent on the very furry white one.

Incredibly, Bitey Boy possessed an uncanny array of tricks. He loved attention. The more the better. 'Scood him up' or 'skitch 'im up' was a reference given by Steve that entailed a lot of grabbing, sock tugging, throwing, patting and growling. There was a conflict with this however, for whenever Bitey got too much of it, he turned into something else entirely. In a split second he decided that he no longer wanted this much attention. So, he became Bitey by name and Bitey by nature.

Another special talent was begging. This was cute for about five minutes, after which we were very annoyed at our friend for teaching him this while we were away one weekend, even if he had a square bottom and was built for it. The years that followed were filled with endless begging opportunities. 'Oh he's so cute, give him just a little scrap.' 'How adorable. Does he like cherries?' On one occasion, he returned from visiting grandma at least 2 kilograms heavier.

Amazingly he did survive to a ripe old age regardless of the cherry pips, however there is one legacy which still haunts us today.

Even though Bitey was a reasonably small dog, he had the uncanny ability to open the fridge, fossick through the shelves, find the leftovers that were reserved for dinner, empty the container and replace it in exactly the same place. Empty. Truly remarkable.

Even more remarkable was how the ghost of Bitey managed to do the same thing. Bitey was an incredible animal on so many levels.

Four Seasons in One Day

That was part of the advertising slogan that was Melbourne. Don't leave home without your jacket or umbrella because even though the sun is now shining with a perfect blue sky and 20 degrees, anything could happen. Those in the know knew that anything could indeed happen. That's one of the things we instantly loved about Melbourne – the uncertainty.

One of the first things Steve did was purchase a three-quarter length woollen coat from a shop in Elizabeth Street which specialised in keeping men walking the pavements warm. The city is laid out in a grid formation of streets which almost channels the winter weather to form wind tunnels. It's nothing to see groups of people huddled together, bent forward against the howling force, wrapped from head to toe with caps, gloves and scarves tied fast, blinking cold tears against the bracing wind. It's so good to be alive!

Melbournians are very outdoor types and even though winter can be hibernatory by nature, you will always see some die-hards riding their bikes against the wind, running around the park or driving somewhere for something to do. If we're not actually going somewhere, we're planning where or what to do next. We are busy people and simply love being active. Picnics in the park, children running around the playground, shopping, entertaining, meeting friends at cafés and restaurants, driving, riding, walking, running. No matter what the activity we're into it ... and then of course there is sport.

Most weekends comprise sport. We *love* it. AFL football in particular is a topic on most people's lips. It's a rare breed of person who doesn't have a team they follow or at least know what is going on with the competition ladder.

Geelong of course is the only team worth barracking for. It does come with a warning in our household however, as eardrums have exploded when umpires seem to continually make the wrong calls. Even earplugs do nothing to protect the blasts of retribution that bounce around our walls and into the surrounding neighbourhood. Dogs are rendered barkless in this situation and a friend always messages me around this time and enquires about my wellbeing and ears. A good time to go for a walk maybe? And miss the game? A huge dilemma.

Football, along with sport of any kind, is the glue that binds Melbournians together. We are fanatics. Winter is bearable because we can snuggle into the couch and enjoy the game each night now from Thursday to Sunday.

We used to look forward to Friday night footy and the commencement of the weekend at a time when games weren't televised as much as they are now. Football marked the end of the working week and was something to look forward to. Often there'd be a meat pie with tomato sauce and glass of red wine to wash it down. So many people supported their teams come rain come shine by travelling to wherever their teams played. We, however, were TV supporters and loved it just the same.

If there were no games being televised, then the rest of the time was spent listening to programs analysing the play and tactics of the game. Marngrook Footy Show was a definite favourite. Being an Indigenous program and slightly left of centre, the panel were made up of past players and coaches with guest players from current teams being interviewed. It was clever because they weren't allowed to show current footage due to ownership rights, but instead the conversation was lively and mostly about the actual game and players, rather than other commercial shows, where commentary was more about the presenters and their past achievements. They also showed past play footage to make a point. Very entertaining.

Football History – City/Country

Football was first played over 123 years ago. Teams represented the area or suburb they trained in and created a sense of community in the playing of sport. Often families supported the same team over generations and passionately followed anything that related to that team. Wearing the colours, making banners, singing the team anthem, collecting player swap cards and finding out anything possible about the players, coach and tactics of how they would win the premiership come September. The dream of the win.

The oldest clubs in Australia are Geelong (1858) and Melbourne (1859). Port Adelaide saw the light and founded their football club in 1870. It's engrained in our DNA. We can thank our Indigenous ancestors, as it was their game called Marngrook that was adapted by a guy called Tom Wills who grew up around where this was played.

Tom, his cousin Henry Harrison, and a couple of mates

MOVING ON

Hammersley and Thompson were bored Aussie cricketers who tapped into their inner athletic selves and created the football game to keep themselves fit in winter before the cricket season recommenced.

The first documented football match was in Richmond paddock in 1858 with 26 players.

Today, Melbourne's sporting precinct sits proudly by the picturesque Yarra River where many stadiums celebrate anything from soccer, cricket, AFL football, rugby and major touring artists from around the world.

You can enjoy a relaxing river cruise along the Yarra after your team wins at the Melbourne Cricket Ground (MCG) located in Yarra Park, stop off at Federation Square or the Arts precinct nearby to check out an exhibition, enjoy a bite to eat at any of the award-winning restaurants that line it's shores, or simply head to Southbank to take in the impressive views at sunset.

It's easy to wile away your time wandering through the many gardens and parks that surround all these precincts, and busloads of tourists can be seen taking photos of the Princess Bridge which connects the CBD with Arts centre, the iconic Arts centre Spire near the gallery and the many market stalls that line the boardwalk.

Melbourne has grown into a lively, vibrant city, becoming an epicentre for sport, art, food and entertainment; something our parents could never have imagined, because for their generation life was simple – but their life stories highlighted how some fundamental things would always remain the same.

City Footy

Steve's mother was a very passionate Fitzroy supporter and as a girl she would go to every game with her family, which included brothers, sisters, parents, cousins and any stragglers who had nothing better to do.

In those days television had only just come onto the scene and not every family was fortunate to possess such a luxury, so going to the game was a ritual and necessary to keep in touch with what was going on. A way of connecting to something outside your own small world.

Football was one of the few reasons for large numbers of people to congregate for a single purpose, other than dances or perhaps church.

Life seemed much simpler then. The week revolved around work, family, extended family, a few friends, church and sport. It was a place to meet with like-minded people and a chance to let off some steam as Steve's father used to say. Being quite a vocal South Melbourne supporter himself explained why the earplugs were required in our own household.

There was a wonderful story about Steve's grandad and friend waiting until three-quarter time to front up at the

Fitzroy grounds in their oversized trench jackets and boots, attempting to impersonate either security or police to gain free entry. Times were tough after the 1930s Great Depression and money tight for a decade after the Wall Street Crash, so you had to be creative to not only survive but to manage to enjoy something of normal life.

This story of struggle morphed into many different versions over the years, but the overall cheeky Aussie ingenuity and laughter that accompanied it were worth every embellishment.

Steve's mother had been known to yell from the boundary of a country game and actually throw her handbag at a player who was supposedly responsible for hurting her young son.

'Don't you hit my boy like that! Leave him alone or you'll have me to answer to!' A very different image to the one of her serenely and happily playing the church organ week in and week out. Abide With Me and Amazing Grace seemed to hold very different meanings.

The game. A truly remarkable thing.

It can stir emotions that you would never expect and from people you would never expect. All ages, types, sizes. All races, all denominations and backgrounds. All people young and old. All people from around the world.

Sport is a powerful thing.

Country Footy

My childhood football experience was very different in country Victoria, which hosted many football games and teams. Small regional townships such as Vinifera, Sea Lake and Manangatang had little more than a corner store, a post office or maybe a pub if they were lucky, but they most certainly had a football team and oval. If they didn't have an oval, they shared one.

Going to these games was such fun. All the family would cram into the old Holden sedan JPC988 equipped with rugs, cushions, thermos of hot tea and sandwiches. As many cars as possible would park around the boundary of the oval for prime position, all facing the inside. This unique rite of passage meant everyone had to be dressed, packed and ready to leave very early that morning to get there and claim their sacred piece of ground. Often as kids we'd be so excited we couldn't sleep the night before. This would work against me in a major way, as there were many times when the second half of the game was lost because I'd nodded off unable to keep eyes open any longer.

If the weather was good there'd be the rug on the grass or mud next to the car. If wet and cold the car windows would be fogged up, condensation running down the inside with us kids constantly bickering about not being able to see. Dad would bring a potato and rub it on the front windscreen as this had magical properties that somehow stopped the rain directly in front of him. That was his story anyway. It did seem rather strange to me, but I wasn't one to argue things I didn't understand. I was more interested in other more satisfying ways potatoes could be used.

Sometimes if we were very lucky or very good or very lucky and good, we would be allowed to share a bag of hot, steamy, soggy chips with loads of salt and tomato sauce dripping all over us. This was Heaven, potato at its best. This didn't happen very often, but when it did it was almost the highlight of the day, along with watching Dad madly beep the horn and flash his lights for every goal in our favour or for every poor umpire's decision.

It was at one of these games that I first realised that the game of footy was complex. The ball was always moving, either by handball or kicking and players were constantly banging into each other, throwing each other around, yelling out and swearing a great deal. The ball was slippery in the wet and bounced strangely due to its unusual shape. Sometimes it went completely in the opposite direction to where it was kicked, and goals in the centre of the white posts were strangely hard to get, even when the player was kicking from directly in front.

Often the most spectacular goals were made in the most tricky circumstances. I'd seen one goal kicked when the player had been thrown to the ground and yet somehow he'd swivelled his body and put boot to ball backwards landing a perfect goal.

It was unpredictable.

It was wild. It was in total contrast to my normal life.

No one in my family spoke about the swearing. In fact I wasn't exactly sure whether the words were bad, as I'd never heard them before. The worst thing I'd ever heard was my dad yelling at my brothers to 'get inside, and get inside ... now!'

There was something about 'darn those boys' or 'for goodness sake ... give me strength'. It didn't matter what dad said, we all knew exactly when we were in strife and going beyond that point was something we didn't want to test out.

The boundaries were very clear.

Sometimes in life we can be doing the same things week after week and then all of a sudden it's like the light shines from somewhere above and something dawns clear. You see something for the first time. That's exactly what happened.

It was half-time and both teams had huddled together in the centre of the field slightly apart, but even so you could hear the players and coaches urging the team to their win in the third quarter. Tense. Anything was possible. Go for it boys!

The umpire blew the whistle, teams in position, the bounce of the ball. The tap was good, the ball landed well and before you knew it went down the corridor, three kicks, two passes and a goal. Just like that.

The goal umpire in his white coat was a favourite of mine. He had a special air of importance about him. I'd seen white coats before at the doctor's surgery and the pharmacist wore one, so I knew he was a man of authority.

It was a goal, so he stood erect, legs apart and pointed two fingers emphatically in front, sometimes bending forward, sometimes jerking the air to make it more obvious.

Then he rushed to take a white flag from both goal posts and flapped them around in a flurry of swirling movements, rolled them up and popped them back as if nothing had happened.

The spectacle was fantastic. Magic.

Maybe it was where we were parked on this day. Maybe it was the light reflecting off the wet grass and squinting into bursts of sunshine. Maybe the gust of wind that blew the flags almost out of hand was the reason … but suddenly I looked away. Something I had never done before.

And there and behold at the other end of the oval was another goal umpire waving his flags at the same time.

What? What on earth? I looked from one end to the other, backwards and forwards, backwards and forwards almost giving myself a whiplash. How could this have escaped me before? Double the excitement.

It was at this defining moment that I decided I needed to take better notice of things. I hated to imagine what else I'd missed out on because I simply hadn't seen it.

This was a puzzling and frightening thing to consider, and something I definitely needed to speak with Mrs Ubergang's cat about, and as soon as possible.

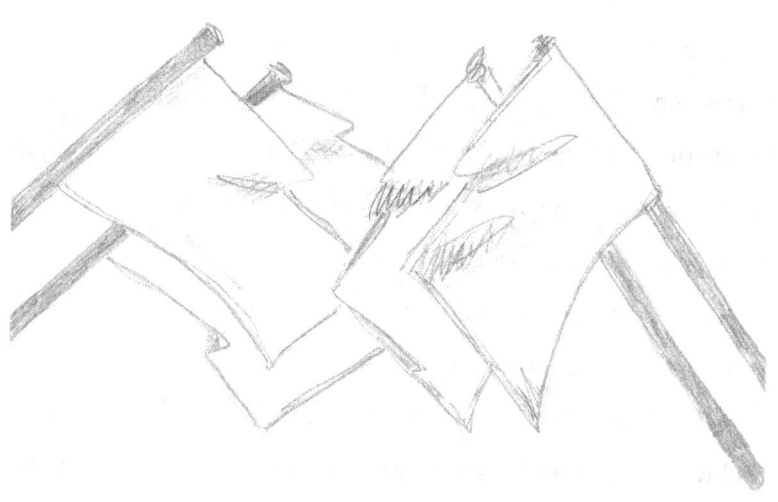

CURRENT DAY

CHAPTER 4

Current Day

Next to sport, Melbournians love coffee. This affair provokes a conversation which is very different to that of sport because it is very individual, and every person who drinks coffee has their own taste, preferences, ideas and opinions about it.

It's not broadcast on TV like sport and there aren't shows every night that discuss the virtues of making the perfect coffee, but discuss it we do. A lot. It's very important to be in the know of any new café in your area as they may have perfected a different brew. This doesn't mean that you would ever be disloyal to your favourite café or barista, it just means that you're up with the latest and got the vibe of the bean.

There's a health benefit of course. Caffeine is a known stimulant and can enhance both the brain and physical activity. Steve loves coffee. It would be dangerous to put a line up before him and ask which is his first love.

In no particular order, football, coffee, iPhone, coffee, football, iPhone, coffee, iPhone, coffee, iPhone, iPhone, iPhone are a few things that come to mind, repeating in their own lovely rhythm. Very dangerous territory indeed, best not to go there.

There are so many varieties and types of coffee that a barista must practise for years to perfect their craft. It doesn't matter whether they are seen wearing a leather cross-over apron in the coolest café or a beanie and check shirt in the corner store – if they can make the latte with the exact level of froth, the right colour and mouth texture, hot and smelling of heaven then they have graduated to Coffee God status and will attract patrons from far and wide.

It can be anything these days. It makes the scene in Steve Martin's film LA Story where everyone around a restaurant table all ordered a drink in a variety of complex requirements finishing 'with a twist of lemon' or some incantation of a twist seem like a very funny joke.

Today that same joke requires low fat, fat, soy milk, almond milk, latte, short, long, double shot, flat white, cappuccino, piccolo, macchiato, espresso, drip, filter with milk on the side.

CURRENT DAY

By the time you've ordered your 'extra hot, double shot, skinny latte with extra milk on the side', the people behind you have wilted and faded into oblivion.

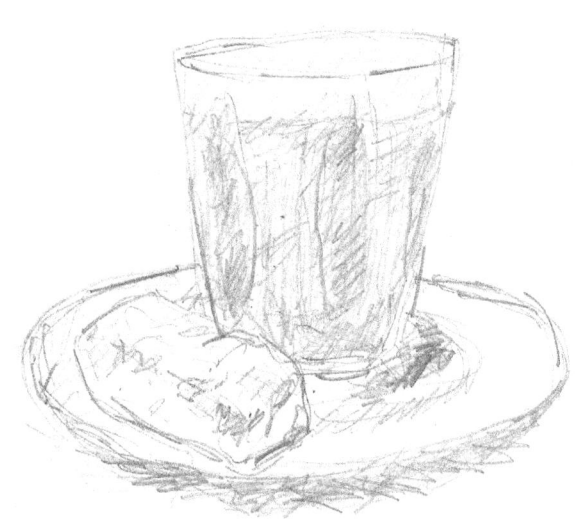

Coffee Ice Cream

Ingredients:

2 cups cream

6 teaspoons instant coffee

1 tablespoon hot water

4 egg whites

¾ cup caster sugar

Pinch of salt

Method:

Beat cream in a medium sized bowl until it has soft peaks and put in fridge to stay cool.

In a glass or jug dissolve instant coffee in 1 tablespoon of hot water.

Beat egg whites in a large bowl with a pinch of salt until stiff peaks form.

Slowly add caster sugar in a stream until egg whites are combined, white and glossy.

Now gently using a spoon, carefully add in batches the whipped cream to the egg white mixture. Don't overdo it; keep it light by not overworking the mixture!

Finally, fold in coffee. Again, be very careful to incorporate gently and as little as possible.

Spoon contents into a container and freeze. Place a folded tea towel on the bench and bang the container a couple of times to get rid of any air bubbles in the ice cream mix.

CURRENT DAY

Serve:

Scoop ice cream into bowl and top with raspberries or strawberries.

Great served between two Anzac biscuits and squashed together as a sandwich.

Make an iced coffee with milk and add coffee ice cream for a double caffeine hit.

Just have it by itself in a cone. Yum!

Note:

Makes 1.5 litres. Serves approximately 8 people.

Will keep for up to a month if you're lucky.

Best to allow a couple of days to really freeze well.

How many coffees are too many?

There's much debate around this. The medical perspective is that an intake of four cups per day is a safe amount. But perhaps the question should also relate to how those cups affect the actual person and in turn, those around them.

There's a coffee barometer that I have applied to Steve over time. What first appeared to be mild enthusiasm, soon developed into a wide-eyed expression of engagement. The stage after cup four was a bit of pacing around and exaggerated arm movements. The finale was where I could only catch the gist of whatever was speedily being said. Words and ideas tumbled out of Steve at a rate where there was no time to respond either with a nod, eyebrow lift or eye blink. Simply watching the lips in complete awe was enough to focus on at this point.

The reality was clear.

In this state, there was no expectation on his part for any kind of involvement from me. It was enough to bear witness, to observe and not lay comment to the uplifting flow of content that eight cups of coffee could bring. A sigh was heard throughout the neighbourhood. Palpitations are also a by-product of caffeine.

Work had been stressful and working long hours had caused some health concerns for Steve. He had always worked long hours and carried the load stoically. Something was now different. Certainly, age has an impact on how our bodies

CURRENT DAY

cope with the stresses of life and in particular our working life. Expectation also carries its own banner and Steve was particularly tough on himself in this regard. He carried this banner high. A heart attack was not something he wanted on his list of achievements.

Sometimes a miracle can happen, and for some unknown reason it came through a personal trainer that Steve had engaged to assist with some of this stress. It was somewhere between the squatting, jumping, running, panting and stretching that it was agreed that he would benefit from a check-up with his doctor. The second miracle occurred when he informed me that he had seen a GP and had a thorough check-up. He was absolutely fine. All good. Nothing wrong. Case closed.

It was some time after this that I observed there had been a marked change in him. Things had settled in some way. The air was not so hot-wired and conversation went both ways. After reducing coffee to under four cups a day Steve's life had taken a very deep breath and exhaled.

I will be indebted to this trainer forever, as a third miracle soon followed the second. I had accompanied Steve for a few sessions to encourage him to stick with the program and was surprised to find how much I enjoyed the process.

'Honestly, why don't you consider doing some study and taking up the profession? You'd be a natural … and it's such a good way to help others … I think you could do it.'

This young personal trainer planted the seed, and also believed without a shadow of doubt that I could achieve it. Without realising it, he had changed the course of my life. I was still singing at Crown Casino at night but had spare time during the day, and so it began.

I had no idea that the body I'd taken for granted contained so many cells, muscles, ligaments, tissue, fibre, systems and complex modes of operation. It was like learning a completely new language and somehow reminded me of the study completed for my musical career. I would need to be patient. This was an entirely different field and would take time to learn.

I soon swam in information and found the only way to make sense of the complicated terminology was to sing it. Strange and bizarre choruses surrounding the connective tissue of the glutes and their insertion points echoed through our apartment. Steve endured many interesting adaptations to the familiar songs in my repertoire. Times had definitely changed, and we wondered what the future might be.

It's funny how life's twists and turns can lead to unexpected places. From any position in time it's hard to imagine what the future may look like or where you may fit in it.

My personal training business began with one client.

Twenty years later, the rest is now history.

CHAPTER 5

Young Love

Steve and I had been best mates since we first met at high school. Growing up together in a small country town meant that there was always something to do. There was never a thought of being bored, it was sport, sport, sport, both in school and after school.

If you weren't involved in sport there was definitely something wrong with you. There had to be a really good reason why you weren't involved and a letter from a parent was needed to excuse your absence.

Steve was pretty sporty. He played footy for the local school team and liked competition tennis, which he played most weekends. He was good at anything he put his hand to.

Things came easily to him, he was bright and was ahead of his class, quick to finish work and didn't need to slog away at homework to keep ahead of the game. This meant that his free time could create opportunity.

There had been a few trips to the principal's office. Nothing done was harmful, however locking someone in the fire hydrant cupboard was not something that was on the school's curriculum and warnings were given.

He had an odd assortment of mates that made up a pack of five or six depending on who was around and what was happening. They were all different but somehow it was their shared sense of humour for the obscure and slightly wacky or some would say abstractly creative that meshed them together. They made their own fun and strangely three of them shared the same name.

They went camping on farms, fishing and hunting rabbits. They wrote and directed movies, mostly about themselves and their adventures. They made objects that no one could make out, sang songs and generally explored everything they could in the freedom that was country living.

It was boys one end of the school quadrangle and girls at the other. Never the two should meet. But as luck would have it the music department was a thriving enterprise in the school and so, when productions of *Godspell* or *Joseph and His Amazing Technicolour Dreamcoat* and *No Flies on Jack* were performed it became the forum for the opposite sexes to unite.

It was during the rehearsals of *No Flies on Jack* that I looked down from the fairy swing dangling in the rafters and noticed a very handsome, angry-looking young boy playing bass with the backing band. It was a musical, and the very clever music teacher had written it specifically for a very keen and not so keen group of male students to channel their creative enthusiasm in another way. This event changed the landscape of the world as we knew it.

Without me realising it, Steve had often glanced up into the rafters to keep an eye on Tinkerbell, and so the love affair began with Steve looking up and Tinkerbell looking down.

I also had a pack of girlfriends, with a nucleus of four. Not wanting to be outdone by the boys, we were also very keen to explore what we could and to prove we were up to the challenge, even though we never had the same freedom that the boys enjoyed.

There was a camping weekend. Three days staying on a friend's farm near the Wakool River. We had borrowed a tent and anything else we could to be as comfortable as possible and were driven to the location by a parent. There were a few rules. The first was no make-up and no mirrors. This was made for one girl in particular whose idea of roughing it was staying in a five-star hotel. Glamping was not on the radar as yet.

Things were going well. The tent was up, the toilet was dug a few metres downhill near some trees. We'd sorted out the food as to who was doing what and settled into gossip and solving the problems we all seemed to face. A guitar meant that we could sing as loudly as we liked, until losing our voices, we'd go for long walks between getting the fire lit and collecting wood.

Day two it rained. Solidly. We stayed in and wondered whether three days away was being a bit too adventurous? There was no choice however, as there were no phones and so we had to make the best of it.

Waking up the next morning it was freezing with a heavy mist and the ground was slippery with mud. There was a scream. Susan bolted into the tent with panic written all over her face. 'What is it? What's wrong?' Everyone was definitely now awake and worried. We may be tough camping girls but at heart we weren't quite as confident as the boys. Only one of us was involved in Girl Guides and those skills differed greatly to what Cubs and Scouts had to offer.

'There's an animal out there! A huge animal! I was going to the ladies when all of a sudden I heard something and then saw it coming towards me!' She threw the torch onto the nearest sleeping bag and covered her eyes trying not to cry. We were stunned.

What could it be? A cow? Possibly, as it was farming land after all. A stray sheep perhaps?

But huge? After some debate we all decided we had to find out exactly what type of animal it was because the thought of never going to the toilet again or not stepping outside to get the fire going was inconceivable. We couldn't just eat potato chips and we'd freeze to death.

One of the girls, namely the girl scout, was first to peek out the tent flap. She opened it a little wider and we all crowded round to see if there was anything there. Then we all saw it at once. Squeal is not a very flattering word but there was no other way to describe the high pitch noise that came out of that tent. 'Aaaaiieeeeeeeeeee.'

There it was. An overgrown, musclebound lizard stalking around the trees nearby. Its long head and jaw looking side to side as it ambled along, tongue flashing in and out. Its enormous meaty tail thrashing and pounding the ground as it moved, and most scary of all its eyes blinking expectantly in our direction. We shut the tent and looked around for a weapon.

Torch. Toilet paper. Guitar. Esky. And perhaps the mirror that one particular girl had managed not to live without for the weekend. There had to be consensus, that was one of our rules.

Debate was fierce and by the time we'd decided perhaps we could just run at it yelling all at once … it was nowhere to be found. This was a huge relief but also strangely worrisome, so we travelled outside as a group after that. When we relayed the horrifying story to the parent the next afternoon for camp pick up, we were to learn that goannas are docile, unsociable creatures that only enjoy eating insects and other creepy crawlies. So, we weren't on the menu after all.

The story was a good one however and by the time we'd relayed it a number of times the goanna had grown into an enormous monster, much to the delight of the boys. Sadly, for us it only confirmed to them that we were after all just girly girls.

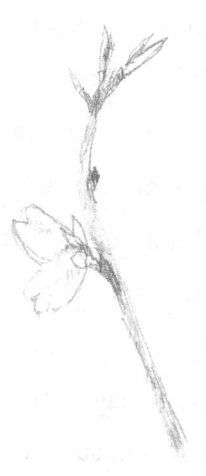

CHAPTER 6

Spring 2019

The weather was at last showing signs of change. The chilly winter wind was being taken over by a milder, softer more considerate breeze that allowed me to take off one of the many layers I'd taken to wearing. Spring in Melbourne is sublime.

Once all the sneezing was over and tissues had been used while waking up, we took long deep breaths. Inhaling the fresh sweet air brought with it a buoyancy, a lightness of step and more smiles of greeting. Hibernation was over and happiness was all around. 'Love is in the air, everywhere I look around' is easy to hum at this time of year.

Not only had the atmosphere lightened but there was a feeling of expectation. Hope. Better days ahead. Spring had magical properties.

Walking around the same inner-city streets brought new wonders. Each day there seemed to be new growth bursting over the fences, buds were getting ready to explode, lavender and camellia scents wafted with each step and trees dressed in cherry blossoms brought tears to the eyes, they were so beautiful. Even dogs sensed that now was the time to get out and enjoy themselves.

They greeted you with tails wagging, jumping for joy if you noticed them. Frankie was in prime position at the gate and ready to receive any number of tummy rubs on offer.

The joy, it is contagious.

Weekends are definitely the highlight of the week. Of course, there's footy to watch and walking around the neighbourhood is always on the list. Shopping at the Prahran Market is really enjoyable as it's a hub of activity and a great place to people watch. Connecting with some of the stall holders over many years has brought with it a comfortable rapport, a smile and chat about anything from the best looking aubergines to when the next grandchild is due.

Prahran Market is Australia's oldest continuously-running food market, established in 1864 it's doors have proudly welcomed customers to the iconic Commercial Road building since 1891. You can buy a coffee from Jasper Coffee, a delicious pastry from a choice of five or more bakeries, a takeaway cheese toastie from Maker and Monger, an assortment of dried and natural organic produce and dinner is made easy with fresh fish, poultry or meat, with numerous delicatessens offering a grazing platter of smallgoods as an even easier alternative to cooking.

It is the market, with it's sense of rhythm, community and connection that has helped me survive the last few years in chronic pain. When even the simplest of activities becomes an effort it's very easy to avoid doing anything that might trigger pain. Just walking slowly to the market was something I had to gradually work toward.

It was a goal that I knew would be challenging but would give so much in return, once achieved. It took months. Steve would help me as I hobbled to the end of the block. I'd be done after a few metres and have to return to bed. Time and again we repeated the same process until gradually the market came into view. I will never forget seeing the façade and realising I was nearly there. I'm sure Steve felt the same. He helped me achieve that goal and now it's something we regularly do together and enjoy. I will never take for granted walking to places I love. Connecting with others and maintaining some semblance of normality is essential for survival.

A CURRAWONG SOMERSAULT

Often without realising it, pain had forced me to retreat physically and in doing so had disconnected me from the simple everyday workings of life that I enjoyed. Dealing with anything that draws a person into themselves can isolate. Lives can be changed in an instant by an event or illness. Often in these circumstances all the surrounding noise and clutter of our lives dissolve into thin air as we are brought back to the fundamentals. The simple things. What really matters.

Simple things have always held meaning for me and this is something I learnt in practice as a young adult. Looking after and caring for older parents was a privilege and a challenge. Sickness and the ravages of decline slowly and systematically took away their simple pleasures, leaving blindness, incontinence and a life unrecognisable.

Dealing with each setback was a lesson in humility and compassion and something which has stayed with me ever since. Finding something small, anything at all to be grateful for when there appears to be nothing, was the most challenging part of caring for my parents. They proved to me that there is dignity and real power in accepting what life throws at you, but not giving in to it.

Being grateful for the simplest of things has meant that I can be very easily pleased and rarely disappointed. Life has a way of giving us what we need at exactly the right time, or in some cases – just in time. I've often received a call or a gentle word of encouragement just when I felt at my wits' end. Time and again I have been reminded that care is a gift given and received. When we give of ourselves we receive far more than we realise. When we shift the focus off ourselves and think of others we can receive so much, if we're open and willing to accept it.

It was Steve who carried most of the produce when shopping. This job fell to him by default because this was one of the forced restrictions of my pain monster. Many adjustments in our relationship had been made over time and many were still a work in progress. Some were obvious in the way something was physically managed, others were much more subtle and complex and to the unassuming eye would be completely undetected, non-existent in fact.

Sometimes things unravelled. Adjusting and changing to accommodate the unknown that was my pain meant that Steve was always the recipient of God knows what. This was difficult, and even though one of his best skills was being adaptable, it was a very different scenario having to navigate what felt like shifting sand under foot. It was impossible for him to know how to react, what to do next and more importantly how to help me. I had turned into someone completely different. He didn't know me anymore or how best to reach out. The combination of hard drugs and constant discomfort from severe back pain rendered me unrecognisable to him. His sad eyes broke my heart. This was the hardest challenge we had ever had to face together and it wasn't going away quickly.

My personal training day had finished early as there had been a couple of clients cancel unexpectedly, so I had made my way home thinking about what lunch might look like. I hate to admit it, but sometimes it was a relief when someone cancelled. Even though I loved my work I still found it very physically demanding and tiring. Some days were worse than others if sleep had been a disaster the night before.

I have made many adjustments so I can still operate my business, most of which replaced my physical involvement with verbal direction.

Using icepacks to numb my back was part of daily life, and being superficially numb really helped me keep going. I took icepacks everywhere and used them constantly. I now tucked two of them into my underwear and made my way home for lunch.

Lunchtime was fairly consistent. I would make Steve a wrap of some description the night before, poached chicken, spinach, grated carrot, boiled egg, avocado and either mustard or mayonnaise. His preference usually involved meat of some type so to mix it up and add an element of surprise he'd sometimes find sliced lamb or ham with olives, capsicum, coleslaw, pine nuts and lettuce. You'd be right to think that we both enjoyed food.

SPRING 2019

Looking in the fridge was a challenge. There was always a lot going on with stacks of things on top of other things. Jars, containers, herbs, eggs, meals that were waiting to be cooked and others that were in transition, half used and soon to be reincarnated into another completely different concoction.

You could juggle things around all day and not achieve any more space than what was started with. The empty containers that Bitey, our departed dog, still managed to leave behind only added to the confusion, but always brought a smile.

It was a rare time when I allowed myself to put tidiness and godliness to one side. Carefully shuffling through the contents, I found a boiled egg, a carrot, some stuffed red peppers, olives, tuna and spinach leaves. Perfect. The courtyard at the rear of the apartment was beckoning with the sunshine already hitting the white marble of the outdoor table. Spring at last.

I was cutting up the carrot and heard a splash. To my delight the little honeyeaters had returned. A number of years ago two lovely little birds had discovered the birdbath.

They liked nothing better than to dart in and among the three slippery elms at the rear of the yard and then plunge in and out of the bath in a blink of an eye. When this happened, I was careful not to blink so I didn't miss anything. They were adorable little things.

Our courtyard by apartment standards is certainly not large, but there could be nothing more that could be added to the green space. Every square inch had a purpose and plants overlapped herbs, overlapped flowers, overlapped veggies all sitting under the watchful gaze of three slippery elms, one cumquat and a stunning Japanese maple which held pride of place close to the lounge room windows.

I had become attached to these birds. They had no idea how much I looked forward to seeing them. Their arrival was noted twice a day in normal conditions, approximately 11 in the morning, which I'd often missed due to work commitments, and between 4 and 4:30 in the afternoon. This was the time I would look forward to each day.

Each year for the past seven years these birds would visit, like clockwork except for daylight savings, which confused things a little. If summer was unusually hot, they'd drop by more often either for a quick bath or drink, their little beaks open, trying to cool down.

But the most marvellous thing was that each year there was an addition. They'd swoop in together; one took pride of place at the bath itself and waited, while another flittered around the courtyard being watched from above by another sitting in the trees above. They worked together, taking it in turns to dive in and out so quickly it made me giggle. They were athletic dive-bombers. No sooner had they dunked into the water than they were out and up the trees, hopping and flapping, preening and chirping.

On one such occasion I was stunned to count five little birds in total. That was a good day. Recently however I'd noticed that they hadn't been to visit and wondered why. Perhaps all the cranes, taking down large trees and building going on outside had caused them to move to safer territory? There had also been a lot more larger birds in the area.

Crows were by no means a favourite. They were many and could be heard early in the morning trying to clear their throats. Time and again they'd croak.

I couldn't help but wonder whether they would ever succeed and actually make a nicer song to listen to. It was the rubbish they were after, and all the building going on around us provided a feast.

White cockatoos were also another large bird that seemed to fly in en masse. They announced their impending arrival from miles away and then you'd have no doubt when they had finally landed in your neighbourhood. They were stunning to see in the sky, white wings spread wide and yellow beaks squawking over the top of each other. Deafening but exhilarating at the same time.

Only a few weeks ago I had witnessed a rare collision of the two species. An aerial display of squawking, swooping, chasing and dive-bombing was seen as they fought to protect the rights of the tall pine tree kernels that were breakfast.

Three cockatoos flew alongside a crow and ushered it convincingly to another area away from the main flock. It went on and on until surrender and breakfast resumed for the victors. The mess on the footpath underneath was the only evidence.

With the lunch bowl now ready I grabbed my mobile phone and started to make my way through the dining area towards the courtyard. Only a matter of steps in a compact apartment, when I suddenly stopped in my tracks. Time suspended and I held my breath.

There was a bird. I didn't know this one.

Something made me smile.

It was long and slender, greyish in colour and squinting, I could just make out some lighter flecks on its wings. 'Damn, I'd forgotten my glasses!' This was something that Steve constantly felt the need to remind me of. 'Why don't you just wear them? … Instead of always hunting for them?'

Oh yes, he was right, of course he was. I knew I'd have to give in to it sometime soon. I'd have to admit defeat and be yet another step closer to becoming my mother. I just wasn't quite ready to go there. Me stubborn? Never!

4:31 pm it happened. The bird had been perched on the wrought iron seat surveying the land and taking note of its surroundings. Then in a beat it hopped to the lip of the birdbath, looked down at the water, looked to either side, turned its back to the water and then flipped backwards into the bath and out. Wings flapping and making honking noises until it found its place back to the starting position. This was fantastic!

Time and again it flipped. Somersaulting from different positions but always a backflip.

As confidence grew the level of difficulty increased and before I knew it I was laughing so hard there were tears running down my cheeks. This was an event to remember!

Sniffing and laughing at the same time I watched it fly up into the tree and beyond while I kept still, in wonder, not wanting the moment to end. I ventured out into the courtyard and looked around my oasis. It was a special place, and I'd often thought it softened the harshness outside that was city life.

The concrete, the pavements, the cars, noise and pollution, but now I realised my courtyard was something quite different. It meant something more. It was the life blood of the bird community and a place where they could find sanctuary. A place to explore, find something to eat, refresh and quench their thirst. A safe place.

But best of all it was a place where they could let loose, dive and flap, somersault and be creative – to find and be their own bird.

A CURRAWONG SOMERSAULT

There have fortunately been many times where I would casually say to Steve, 'Now don't turn quickly but just look to your right and you'll see our friend.'

Countless times he has tried to slowly reach for his phone, even positioning it on a stand at the window ready to press video at the next showing, but clever as Steve is, he is always outwitted by Flippy bird as we have now lovingly named him.

And yes 4:30 pm does seem to be significant in the bird world clock. Flippy bird does his best acrobatics at this time and perhaps it is this extravagant behaviour that has pushed the little honeyeaters to the later 5 pm time slot. Either way the parade is welcome and the back-to-back performance is enjoyed by all who witness it.

CHAPTER 7

With Challenge Comes Strength

'It's only for a year' says Steve, his face animated and wary at the same time. I can remember every detail of that day. I stood one side of the kitchen bench and he the other.

He was leaning on the stool and I had to lean on the bench in case I found myself on the floor.

Work had been sporadic for Steve, his industry had shrunk and Melbourne no longer housed the many global advertising agencies of the past. There had been mergers and acquisitions, shuffles and reshuffles. Times had changed in the advertising industry and now Steve was left to ponder his future and how he could survive it.

He had engaged in additional media studies and web-related work in the hope that diversifying would open some opportunities and doors. Never in my wildest dreams did I imagine the door would be that of a plane that would take him and his expertise to the other side of the world.

In the past there had been business travel for Steve; a day here and there for work or a week or two if required. This was a very different scenario. Uncharted territory with no point of reference. 'An opportunity too good to pass up', 'Once in a lifetime', 'What else am I going to do? There are no other options on the table', 'I'll come back as often as I can' ,'You'll get better and soon be able to join me' and 'The money will take away some of the stress'.

All of the arguments were valid. There was nothing to be said as an interview was scheduled in the United Emirates. 'Let's see what happens, we have nothing to lose going through the process.' So many conflicts. So little time. I was trapped between wanting Steve to be happy and find his place again and not wanting him to leave.

His confidence had slipped away and I knew he needed this. My confidence along with my heart however was now packed neatly in his baggage. This was the first time we had ever lived apart. Steve's business world was opening up with exciting possibilities overseas. My world was retracting even further as I considered how I would survive alone.

Alone with pain. Comfort can be found from unexpected places. You don't realise what you carry with you in your memory bank until it's required. Childhood images came back to me as if they knew I needed to be reminded of simple carefree days.

Childhood Sunday Lunch

Every Sunday was the same with only a few variations to the theme. There was Sunday School for the kids at the local church, followed by running around the church grounds while the adults talked at the front or inside the hall where tea and coffee were provided.

We all wore our Sunday best which comprised pressed pants, shirt and tie for my brothers and tights, hair ribbon, black or red shiny shoes and a dress with prickly underskirt for me.

We'd run around until completely exhausted and then walk along the high brick fence that was the boundary to the church grounds. That's if you were big enough to get on it, of course. It was a wonderful day when you found that at last you could heave yourself up and balance one foot in front of the other along the narrow ledge. Once you were able to do it you then had to be careful not to be seen doing it, as it wasn't the most lady-like thing to do in your Sunday best.

Once home everyone was as quick as sticks to get out of their best clothes and into something much more comfortable ready for lunch. Sunday lunch was either at home together with our Nanna and Grandad or over at their place a few blocks away.

I was often in the way of my brothers. Trying to keep up and be a part of what they were doing was all I wanted to do. Truth be known I didn't really think much about being a girl or doing what girls do and even though my mother made outfits for my dolls so I could dress them up, I much preferred running up and down the dirt embankments at the back of our house, or jumping in the irrigation channel playing hide and seek among the reeds. Probably for this reason I often found myself having lunch with my parents at Nanna and Grandad's. The boys had been excused. They were older. That's what happened.

One such Sunday we were all seated around the dining table and Nanna had just taken away the dishes and was in the kitchen getting ready to serve dessert. This was a treat as she was an excellent cook and often made cakes, flans, sponges and slices. Anticipation is such an amazing thing for a child, and I could hardly wait to see what Nanna had in store.

I was seated next to my mother with my grandad at the end of the table. He was old. He seemed much older than Nanna even though they both had white hair and wore cardigans. As I looked at him, I noticed he was nodding off, he was actually having a nap at the table. This was something I had never seen before but thought perhaps he too was thinking about dessert.

WITH CHALLENGE COMES STRENGTH

Nanna arrived with the jam and sponge tart and placed the servings in front of everyone, giving Grandad a gentle nudge when no one was looking. It was then that my eyes widened as I watched him put a huge dollop of mayonnaise on his dessert instead of cream. I was mesmerised and held my breath. He ate it. Every single mouthful without a word.

I made a mental note to ask Mum and Dad about that on the way home but was then distracted when Nanna asked if I had started ballet yet? This was high on my wish list and Nanna knew how much I adored anything which required a tutu.

After doing a little pirouette or two around the dining room and striking a pose for her, she came and gave me a hug. Then as she rubbed my arms she said, 'Don't worry about the hair on your arms, dear. It's a sign of strength and will disappear as you get bigger.'

This was a problem I had not even been aware of, let alone considered, and as I looked from my Nanna to my father and back again, I realised that my father had an enormous amount of hair on his arms and his eyebrows were bushy and unkempt. I burst into tears and declared 'I didn't want to be strong if that was the case'. I loved my father very much but there was no way I wanted to have his hairy arms or eyebrows!

Mrs Ubergang's cat would surely know something about the subject. Getting home was the most important thing to happen next, dessert was a thing of the past.

A CURRAWONG SOMERSAULT

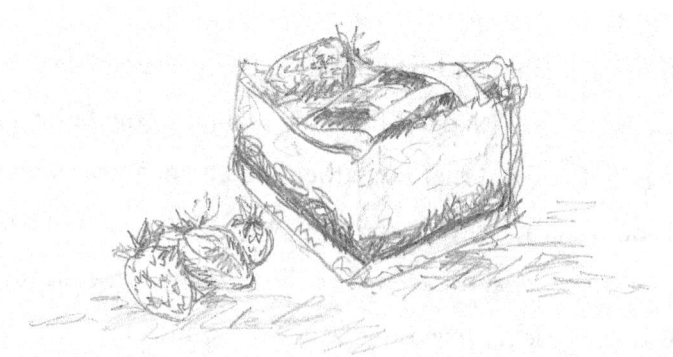

CHAPTER 8

Farewell

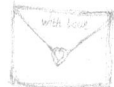

The bags along with a pushbike were collected and sent ahead. The family had all said their goodbyes with a number of dinners and get-togethers; no one really able to say exactly what they were thinking or feeling but the vibe was positive and supportive. 'It may not work out, let's see how things go', 'We can always Skype', 'Keep us in the loop', 'He's just like his father and needs another adventure'.

I couldn't bring myself to wave goodbye. I couldn't guarantee that I'd be able to hold together the emotion that was sitting front and centre in my chest. The weight was almost too much to bear. Instead I left a goodbye message on the kitchen bench, so that at 5 am he would find it and have something of me to take with him. Something tangible, something real, something from my heart.

I'd rather remember the night before and the special meal we'd shared together, the smiles, the hopes, the expectation of better days ahead. The last thing I wanted to do was imprint a sad memory for us both.

I lay silently in bed and listened, it was the normal routine; the shower, rustling around for clippers, shave, a few coughs, followed by more rustling.

Dressing in the bathroom created more noise and then navigating the dark brought with it a swear word as he collided with the door. I held each process along with my breath and committed them to memory. The key rattled and the door closed. I exhaled, turned over and wept uncontrollably. Farewell.

I knew what it was to wait. I had waited before. Young love finds it hard to wait, but strict parents know that if something is real, and love is true, then time and its passing will only make it stronger … or not.

Oh yes, I knew how to wait. I waited five years to marry Steve. We were too young to understand what real love was, my parents thought I was too young to know my own mind and heart. Time passed, as they said it would.

We married young – then promptly moved to Adelaide.

FAREWELL

The next year without Steve was a blur for me. Work as a personal trainer was as it always was. Most of my clients were regulars or had been referred by someone who I had helped in the past, they were men and woman, young and old, who each had a set of different health issues and requirements, unique in every sense of the word. Much of my work was with the physical side of health but I also incorporated the psychological benefits of coaching for positive outcomes. I felt it was important not to give my own opinion to many of the underlying issues my clients presented and working closely with others offered a unique opportunity.

In a safe haven of trust, my clients knew that whatever was said within the four walls not only stayed there, but was received with respect, love and without judgement. I wanted to approach my care from the inside out.

Many of the physical ailments I treated were clearly linked to deeper internal problems, so I attended a variety of courses and became a life coach, training with The Coaches Consortium and also attended Melbourne University completing a Cert. IV Train the Trainer qualification.

I was a stretch therapist and personal trainer, and incorporated all of these components in the program to achieve the result I was looking for. This worked well for my clients and I was rewarded by seeing changes for the better in their lives as well as their bodies. Sometimes I was taken by surprise.

Healing can be unpredictable.

Not only did I feel able to assist their health and wellbeing but more often than not I became the humble recipient of my clients' care and concern in return – something that only time, respect and genuine honesty can provide.

Most of them were aware that Steve was working overseas. Many understood the reasons why and it was nothing for me to find a little parcel of lasagne left on the counter on departure or a bunch of flowers as a little cheer up.

Even though I felt the weight of loneliness creep into my evenings and the shift in physical pain become more and more intense each day, I settled into the routine of work, Skype, lunch, rest, work, Skype, bed.

Initially work was a distraction and I never valued my clients more than during this time. I had managed the back pain as best I could but as time progressed it was getting harder and harder for me to hide it. I was still using icepacks and taking medication as directed but the amount of rest required between clients was increasing and I was starting to struggle with the everyday workings.

Megan, one of my friends, was kindly doing the most strenuous cleaning for me, and family often visited providing a meal and extra support. Something had shifted and the pain was starting to overtake me. My clients were now asking how I was and it was becoming clear I wasn't operating at my usual levels. This was concerning as I prided myself in getting on with it, pushing through and rising above any negative.

Pain will always win.

This was the stand out comment I remembered after my first meeting at the pain management department at the hospital. It kept ringing in my ears as I wept uncontrollably on the hospital bed. The psychologist speaking gently to me waited for me to gain control so they could proceed with their evaluation.

I had never cried like this before. Never in front of someone else. Even though I was totally embarrassed, I was at the mercy of a force beyond my control. I was done.

'Take your time, it's not something you can fight ... take some deep breaths and tell me what would you say to your clients ... if they were dealing with what you are currently?'

Suddenly, amongst the fog in my mind there was a moment, a light, something to hang onto in a dark deep hole.

I'd given my professional life to help others ... what would I say? The right words would always come when they came from the heart ... 'Be kind to yourself ... take a breath ... it's ok to let it go ... oh God ... what's happening to me?'

'This is normal ... what you are experiencing is extreme pain. You were admitted to hospital because of this and you need the right medication and treatment to help you manage it differently … we will be helping you with this.'

'Is there anyone at home who can help you?'

For a second time I lost control. Tears flowed from unimaginable depths.

I could never truly understand why we try and protect those that we love. It had taken all my strength to somehow deflect what I was going through, not wanting to add to the pressure that Steve was under already. He had taken the job overseas and was working hard day and night. He shared an apartment with three others, renting a room to help reduce costs. Everything about his new life in Dubai was alien and I could see the stress in his face and eyes each time we Skyped so I thought that the last thing he needed to know was *my* struggle.

Is being protective being honest? I wasn't sure, the only thing I was sure about was that I needed help. Pain had brought life to a new base. It was raw. It was humbling. It was looking deeply at myself. Facing myself with complete honesty. This was exhausting and very confronting. It seemed as though my life was being driven by forces beyond my control, and instead of fighting with this I needed to learn a different way.

I thought I knew myself fairly well but this was an entirely different level of self-discovery. Feeling out of control brought with it fear. Was I losing my mind as well as control of my body? These were dark thoughts and I had never felt so lost.

The pain clinic and its patients provided shared experiences that cut to the bone, shedding light on untold fears, exposing hidden coping behaviours and exploring the many restrictions pain imposed. It was a safe place to find another way. And even though it didn't seem like it at the time, it was a place that brought about healing and acceptance. Once there was acceptance, the change gradually happened mentally. It wasn't until years after that I could actually see the shifts that had happened to me. It was gradual. Painstakingly gradual. Slowly working with managing pain and myself.

One foot after the next as if back as a young girl on the single brick fence, balancing to stay alive. Patiently and sometimes not so patiently. After nearly two years I was able to recognise myself again, or should I say, another version of myself.

All the while finding the strength from deep within, from somewhere unknown, a pool that could only be accessed with complete honesty. No judgement. No expectation. No fear.

During this time a small voice spoke softly to me. It spoke of reassurance. It spoke of certainty when all else was uncertain. It listened and encouraged. It was the gentle voice of someone I loved dearly and someone I missed. It reminded me to be patient. I listened and realised I was at last learning to be kind to myself.

Nanna Wilson

"When something doesn't work one way you have to find another."
– Nanna Wilson

My Nanna had many pearls of wisdom. At eight years of age I didn't recognise this and as I tried to close the gate to the chook pen, I felt all I was doing was fighting with it and so far, the gate was winning. 'Slow down, dear, and try another way.'

I stopped the pushing and pulling and kicking and pursed my lips. I hated these lessons.

I somehow felt I was so much older than my years. Many of the adults around me often commented on my broad vocabulary, considerate manner or quick thinking.

I found it very frustrating to be wrestling with a gate and for my Nanna to notice. I was embarrassed. I adored my Nanna and only wanted to please her, so looked at the gate closely. It was old of course, with old wooden planks repurposed with chicken wire, screws and rusty nails and a large round iron knocker as a handle that flapped around in the wind when the weather took hold.

I could see the wire was coming apart at the bottom and it really was sitting at an awkward angle. Then it was clear, the bottom was crooked and it was making a trench in the dirt beneath it and the groove was starting to build up.

FAREWELL

In a flash I looked up at Nanna, who was smiling. I bent down and quickly scooped away the dirt, using my hands to pile it up next to the gate. When finished I dusted off my hands and stood looking at the gate. All the while the chickens clucked around it eager to be let out onto the rear grass so I shooed them away, took hold of the handle and after a little tug it opened into the pen amid a flap of wings and squawks. Success.

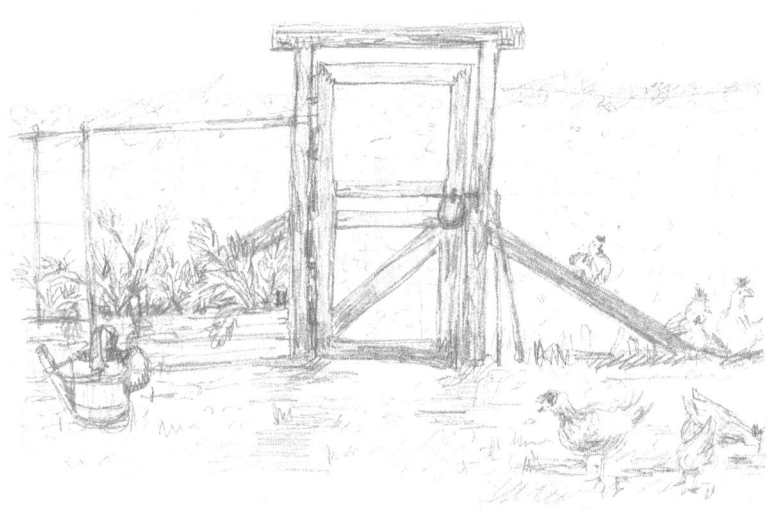

Ginger Fluff Sponge Cake

Ingredients:

4 eggs (room temperature)
½ cup caster sugar
½ cup cornflour
2 tablespoons plain flour
½ teaspoon cream of tartar
½ teaspoon bicarb soda
1 teaspoon cocoa powder
1 teaspoon cinnamon
1 teaspoon ground ginger
1 dessertspoon golden syrup
Pinch of salt

Method:

Set moderate oven 190ºC (170ºC fan forced).

Grease and flour 2 sandwich sized cake tins putting non-stick paper on the base of each.

Sift dry ingredients 3 times.

Gently warm the golden syrup and set aside.

Separate eggs whites, beat with pinch of salt until stiff and forming white peaks.

Gradually add sugar in batches until combined and glossy.

Keep beating, gradually adding egg yokes until light in colour and volume has expanded.

In stages sift in the dry ingredients, gently folding through. Lastly, fold in the golden syrup.

Pour into prepared tins. Cook for 20–25 minutes, until golden and firm to touch.

Cool on baking trays. Ice with either coffee icing and fresh raspberries, or dust with icing sugar to serve.

CHAPTER 9

Cultural Hub

Being adaptable has to be one of the most important things we learn in life. Change happens with or without our consent and time marches on taking us with it for the ride. We plan what we can and loosely work within the things we control, but even the best laid plans can unravel and lead us to unimaginable places, sometimes for the better.

Adelaide had served us both well. Moving to Adelaide meant I could do further studies at the Adelaide University Conservatorium of Music, specialising in jazz notation and improvisation for vocal and pianoforte. Over a 10-year period, I taught pianoforte, singing, performed professionally in the five-star hotel circuit with funk bands Cat's Tango and Blue Indigo, and at the Adelaide Casino and Arts centre, and co-wrote and performed an a cappella show called *Bodies and Souls*, which featured in the Adelaide Fringe Festival.

The musical opportunities I had experienced in Adelaide had provided a broad range of employment both in vocal harmony and a variety of jazz and funk bands, but we embraced the sheer scale of what Melbourne had to offer with open arms.

Steve was a bass player and his playing had to take a back seat while he concentrated on earning a living so that I was able to concentrate on singing as a career instead of working at the same time to make ends meet.

The vocal harmony group *Vocamotion* I had auditioned for and then joined in Melbourne, was entertaining crowds and festivals around Australia, appearing on regular TV shows including Bert Newton's *Good Morning Australia*, and was the platform which helped hone my skills. Without any accompaniment there was nowhere to hide and each of the members were not only multi-talented but were a force in themselves with knockout personalities. I had previously enjoyed playing and singing in clubs and bars in Adelaide but found the raw and entertaining nature of the show they presented both refreshing and challenging.

This completely took me out of my comfort zone, even though I understood and loved harmony I found the intricacy of the arrangements and the way they were delivered a very new experience. Learning 30 songs in two weeks nearly killed me.

It was nothing to drive all night to Sydney for a festival gig, two cars in tandem talking, singing, laughing and sharing stories on the way, stopping for smokes for the smokers and drinks for the drinkers. On arrival the group would stay with friends who over the years had become number one fans and as a result ... good friends.

I can remember arriving in Sydney in the wee hours to be greeted by a couple of equally larger-than-life characters very keen to get the party started. Dr Sid's laugh exploded as he opened the door and his enormous frame matched the laugh and consumed the hallway, amid smells of lamb roast that had been cooking for hours awaiting our arrival. It astounded me just where they all got the energy from, as I was struggling to stay awake and was starting to feel nauseous.

On entering the large apartment one of the guys announced to Cathy, who was seated on the settee, 'Oh Cathy, here we are at last, it's so good to see me!' and quick as a flash the laughing response from Cathy lifting her legs off the floor in front of her, 'Yes Max, it is, even my shoes are pleased to see you!' Such quick wit and at 4 in the morning after travelling so far astonished me, but I knew I'd get on famously with Cathy and her bright red patent leather shoes.

After excusing myself to get some sleep I realised for the first time that not only would it be challenging finding my place in the group, but that they would probably be wondering exactly how they would adjust to this much quieter version of themselves.

It was a restless night, listening to the boisterous conversation snippets and analysis of the new girl and my first real encounter with spending a few hours in the same room with the only other girl in the group. A new and remarkable friendship with Megan was forged over time, regardless of the many sleepless nights endured due to her enthusiastic snoring.

"All good things must come to an end"
– Geoffrey Chaucer, poet, 1380s, Troilus and Criseyde

I had no idea why all things good must end, but end they did. After less than a year the group disbanded amid strange conflicts and misunderstandings of leadership and direction. To the astonishment of most members, our last performance ended up being at The Lemon Tree, an iconic Melbourne haunt for performers and musicians.

To this day I had no idea exactly what happened. Some kind of weird childhood insecurity lurked inside me trying to lay blame on my shoulders, but I couldn't claim it as my own, because the problems within the group had been brewing long before my arrival. I had no clue about these at the time, but over the years that followed I heard pieces of the jigsaw that made sense of the complete picture. I felt sad but also grateful to have worked with such talent.

On With the Show

"From little things big things grow"
– Paul Kelly, songwriter, 1993

Whenever something changes in life, whether it be by design or completely unexpected, there can follow a time of confusion and a general unsettling.

This was the case for me. I had thrown myself shoes and all into the a cappella group and it had consumed me. Now what? I was at a loss. Steve was still working hard and was kind enough to see I needed time to settle and regroup.

Little did I realise that very soon regroup would be literal.

One thing I did know for sure, and that was I wanted to continue working with the other female member, Megan. Putting the snoring to one side, I had found a friend of a lifetime and didn't want to lose that connection.

And so it began, the dream was born. Megan and I plotted and planned over numerous cups of tea and coffee. A new show. A new group. Harmony at its best. High end entertainment.

The thoughts were good ... but what would it look like? We had no idea. What could it be? I had never been able to dream like this before. I had some time, I made a list.

If I could sing anything I wanted to ... what would I choose?

I listened.

If I could name my favourite a cappella singers ... who would they be?

I made another list.

If I could go to any concert featuring clever vocalists ... what would I choose?

I waited.

If I could do anything I wanted ... anything at all ... what would it be?

I went through all the boxes of music stored in the cupboards. I sorted through old records and recordings, listened to concerts and artists, until I was beginning to wonder if inspiration had stayed in Adelaide with the last move. It was the last box of CDs and I was on the floor surrounded by them. I was getting tired and was just thinking a cup of tea may help proceedings and then I saw it, on the bottom of the pile.

'Ah-hah ... there you are,' I smiled. 'I've been waiting for you ... what took you so long?'

With cup of tea in hand, I settled on the sofa and listened to the music which would soon become the basis of a new show.

A Tribute to the Manhattan Transfer would be a show that highlighted our vocal abilities and would need a backing band and two other male vocalists. It would also need to be scripted and the music and arrangements written.

It was a huge amount of work.

It would take time.

It would take commitment.

It was a vision. I could imagine it.

Would anyone else? I immediately rang Megan.

Auditions commenced. Finding two stand-out male vocalists who could tackle this type of vocalisation was now the number one priority.

If they could read music and help me with the vocal scores and musical arrangements, then that would be a major bonus. The band could wait.

I knew it would take time. Everything did, at least everything that was worthwhile. Megan was a rare talent, but she didn't read music as such.

She could follow the note movement up and down to see where things were headed, but this could prove challenging for the complicated harmonies of Manhattan Transfer, and I wondered how this might work. Having done so much study myself over the years, it astounded me how she could manage so well by ear.

With such an amazing voice, Megan had never bothered

with the theory of music because she had an incredible ear and she would laugh. 'It was due to being deaf as a child and having to listen to compensate.'

I was sure she could pick up the tune quickly and find her way around without ever needing to read the music, she'd manage and rise to the challenge, she had spunk.

Her voice ... well that was another story, it was in a class of its own. She wasn't called Megan Mega Star for nothing.

The bass singer was decided. Brilliant. Ben was not only an amazing vocalist and known vocal harmony singer in Melbourne, but he could act, play the piano and also write music. Done.

The search continued and after a few auditions that weren't quite right he announced he knew someone who may be interested.

Nothing could have prepared us for the voice and luckily we were standing against the lounge room wall, because the gentle intonation followed by the full force of what came out of John's mouth simply blew us away.

This talented tenor could sing, act, play piano very well, write music and arrangements and had experience writing script. Perfect.

Writing a show takes time. It's a long process. *I'll Take Manhattan* was loosely scribed onto manuscript as Megan and I welcomed the two male performers.

We worked tirelessly on vocal scores, arrangements, writing the script between songs; imagining how the stage and lighting would work, rehearsing and re-rehearsing all the complexities that go with making a show look effortless.

Even the choreography was painstakingly practised in front of bedroom mirrors until it was perfect, before hiring space at a dance studio to include props and costumes.

I had never before worked with a group of musicians who also wanted to create something so unique. We all shared the vision, we all worked hard. It was a vision of excellence and it was demanding.

Everyone had day jobs of some description to pay the bills as the time slipped by – creativity takes time.

Everyone had other people and family who also needed their attention – creativity can't be rushed.

Everyone was exhausted. We rehearsed after hours, late into the night.

Even creativity was becoming tired of being creative.

No one could say the words. It sat there ... unsaid ... mid-rehearsal. Would we ever succeed?

An idea without a plan is just a wish.

I had seen the band a few times before. Mistaken Identity, a five-piece ensemble, were incredibly talented and could play complex jazz on their ear. I had nothing to lose, and so approached them with the concept.

A CURRAWONG SOMERSAULT

After a few meetings, the dream was sold to them. The rest simply fell into place because when everyone saw them perform at a gig, it was decided they were a perfect fit and we started rehearsals for the show, along with recordings for future promotion.

This was the boost everyone needed.

We had the show, all we needed now were the gigs. I set to work. I contacted agents, set up meetings, rang everyone I could think of and finally found a fellow enthusiast who was the General Manager of the Paul Dainty Corporation. We formed a friendship and very soon gigs were set.

Sometimes life can be strange. For the most part, I had always worked towards something, if *this* is done then *that* can be achieved. It was a constant moving on to the next thing, setting the bar a little higher each time and always working towards the next goal.

I was always optimistic and hopeful, always willing to give it my best shot. This felt different. It was becoming clear to me that much of my professional singing career had been leading to this very point and in some ways it felt like a culmination. This was new territory.

After two years we had created a show with hard work, determination, vision and commitment. I had found like-minded people, now dear friends, who shared music and excellence to achieve something amazing, something from nothing.

Opening Night – I'll Take Manhattan

Nothing more could be done and I looked around the room and smiled at Megan. 'Can you believe it? ... If I had any energy left ... I'd suggest a celebratory drink.'

Megan came over and gave me a hug, 'we did it ... we actually did it.'

We stood there taking in our surroundings. This was the moment we had been waiting for and it was important to let it all sink in. Time as I knew had a way of going nowhere ... fast. Except of course if you're writing a show from scratch.

Mietta, as if on cue, brought over three glasses of champagne to propose a toast. What a wonderful woman, and incredible mind-reader. She'd been the first to support us with a venue, after being approached by our friend at Paul Dainty Corporation. She agreed to supply the venue and dinner and we agreed to entertain the guests. *I'll Take Manhattan* was to perform four nights at Mietta's including dinner and show. It was sold out in the first week. The stage was set.

The boys entered. They were already dressed ready for the performance and were laughing about something. 'Oh there you both are ... we thought we'd lost you ... and on opening night ... what a disaster that would have been ... aren't you getting changed? We'd hate to have to go on without you.'

Megan and I left mid-joke ... 'We were beautiful enough as it was and didn't need much time to put on the finishing touches ... thank you very much.'

It was at this point that we both received beautiful bouquets of flowers from Dr Sid. He apologised he couldn't make it in person, but he knew we'd knock 'em dead!

Tears and a quick retreat – Megan and I needed to get our act together and fast.

The band were playing the overture as the lights dimmed. I stood with Megan and listened. We looked at each other and smiled while the boys paced up and down the hallway outside the room, both restless, both doing their last vocal warm-ups.

I took a deep breath. Well ... this is it, and motioned for everyone to come together.

'Well friends ... we've done it ... we've put in our best. I'm so proud of us ... let's give this crowd everything they hoped to see tonight ... let's knock 'em dead.'

Mietta shook everyone's hands and wished the best of luck. 'It would be wonderful,' she said, 'because we were wonderful.' She opened the door, the announcement was given and our hearts skipped.

Please welcome to the stage ... *I'll Take Manhattan*.

The music soared. The applause deafened.

Lights blinded us as we went through our paces.

I could see a few outlines of people seated around the stage, it was dark but I could see the smiling faces. 'Tuxedo Junction', 'Twilight Tone', 'Spice of Life', 'Java Jive', 'Chanson d'Amore', 'Operator' filled the room. A medley of their songs was woven around a complex story of how Manhattan Transfer met and became the stars they are today.

When it was humorous, people laughed. At times it was sad and there was silence. The music and songs worked their magic. 'A Nightingale Sang in Berkeley Square' brought tears.

'Four Brothers' burst into the room as the finale and the four of us looked at each other as we delivered our lines, eyes bright, smiles broad. With the last flash of light, all the hours of work and heartache faded away amid the roar of applause. Bows and encores, laughter and inexplicable joy.

Everyone received what everyone had hoped.

This night would stay with us for the rest of our lives.

Mietta welcomed us with open arms. She had popped the champagne and quickly ushered the group into a private room. 'Let them wait ... You deserve to enjoy this special moment.'

We humbly accepted the acknowledgement that our hard work had achieved, and without hesitation enthusiastically accepted Mietta's kind offer of an extended season.

Clearing Out

'You're going to have to throw away some of these things, this paperwork is getting out of control,' Steve said. 'Do you want me to start doing it for you?' He was right of course, the boxes and boxes of paperwork were stuffed into not only the second bedroom wardrobe but also all the cupboards at my workplace.

A shiver went through me, because I knew the devastating effects that Steve's cleaning up could produce. This was a threat with ramifications which could cause fallout.

Much of the paperwork was music related – the history of all my piano, theory and ballet accreditations, original songs, manuscripts, musical vocal charts, exams and certificates – and of course *the show*, housed in at least three to four boxes.

The memories associated with writing and performing *I'll Take Manhattan* were precious. Those boxes held so much more than the documentation; the hard work, the planning, the friendships, the time and creative effort, were nothing compared to the joy of performance and satisfaction of pleasing audiences.

We all received so much from the experience and even to this day Megan will celebrate a New Year by viewing one of our performances. It's good to be proud of hard work and a special achievement. I often wondered if more could be done with the show. Could someone else now benefit from using the material? The question remains unanswered although I had considered a lock on the door in case Steve's clean-up ventured beyond a threat.

And then, there was all my parents' final paperwork. Being executor of their estate meant we had to retain all their history for at least seven years.

These had been sitting now for over 10 years. There are some things that seem just too hard to face. Could it be that long? Just the thought alone brings a shudder and a whole range of emotions that are tucked back into their space.

Time and again I had been determined to start the process. I'd purchased a shredder from Officeworks and had managed to cull our out-of-date financials and loose bits of paper stacked in the second bedroom stash, but anytime I opened the wardrobe and looked up at the odd assortment of boxes and then down at the red zip-up overnight bag that contained my mother's few keepsakes I'd promptly shut it and announce, 'Another day.'

On a rare brave occasion I had opened the bag, because I had to pull everything out of the stacked wardrobe to find something else that was needed.

This was a constant source of annoyance for poor Steve. 'There's so much stuff, stacked on more stuff ... when are you going to sort out this mess?'

I couldn't answer Steve because I didn't know the answer.

If I was a bird. I would be a bower bird.

Things held meaning to me. Not all things, but certainly things that were linked with people and places I loved, and sadly for Steve I had a big heart.

Steve on the other hand could live quite comfortably without much at all. That's not to say he didn't appreciate good items, as he had accumulated a huge assortment of bags from travel and he liked nothing better than to sit in his favourite Borge Mogensen vintage chair and doodle away the time on his computer.

But when it came to holding onto things of the past he was very different to me. The most prized possession he had from his upbringing were two tiny wood carvings of elephants minus their tusks that his mother had bought while travelling overseas before she was married.

He remembered playing with them so much that the tusks went missing, so the elephants now sit proudly underneath the lamp and get a polish of oil every time the furniture needs a bit of love.

How can a life be brought down to a bag?

It's easy. Things are quite simple really and as I get older I'm becoming aware of just how simple.

A comb, a box full of embroidery thread and needles, a diary, some handkerchiefs with my mother's initials on them, a worn purse with loose change and a few safety pins, her evening dress with sheer overlay that looked like a floral garden, an old leather-bound hymn book, a bunch of dried lavender, some letters from my grandmother and dad, a Mother's Day card I had made, a jewellery box full of costume jewels and paper clippings announcing family events, engagements and a glasses case with take-away sugar sachets tucked between the glasses.

Very simple indeed.

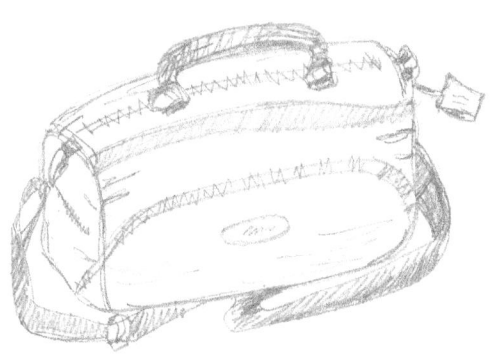

A CURRAWONG SOMERSAULT

CHAPTER 10

Homecoming

A year and a half had passed amid fleeting visits from Steve. It was always wonderful to see him and felt strangely surreal. I found myself in a constant state of flux. Family wanted to see him also and there never seemed to be enough time to accommodate everyone and so it was often a group get-together.

I can remember the first time he arrived earlier than expected. I'd set my alarm for midnight and had put a welcome home sign on the door. I was in bed, now dozing on his side of the bed, something which helped me sleep in some strange way.

I woke with a start when I heard the door rattling and then his greeting as he came up the stairs. 'Poss, poss, poss.'

Never before had I been so glad and startled at the same time.

I flew out of bed – to hell with the back – and wrapped my arms around him. 'Oh my goodness, what happened? You're so much earlier than expected? How wonderful!'

He had managed to arrange a connecting flight and wanted it to be a surprise. That worked! We sat up and shared a cup of tea and talked through his latest news and then, shower, bed. Once there, all I could do was look at him. He was exhausted. Lying next to him I could hear the rhythm of his breathing and the warmth of his body. Home is where the heart is.

Yes Nanna, you were absolutely right and there would be no sleep for the rest of the night for me.

Steve sighed and exclaimed that 'this is the most comfortable bed in all the world' and then asked how I was going? I could no longer hide my turmoil. Amid tears and sobs I somehow let out the months of struggle I had hidden away. The hospital stay, the pain clinic, the loneliness, the pain, the injections, the drugs, the work pressure, of being trapped in a very small space, of missing my best friend and partner.

None of this was actually spoken, but my shaking body expressed the intensity of everything to Steve and he understood the depth of it all. He held me close and shooshed me to sleep. There had to be a better way.

HOMECOMING

Skype saved us. Even though the time difference was an issue at times it was good to see Steve gobbling down his breakfast before he was picked up by his driver because no one walked anywhere in the Middle East; it was 50 degrees in the shade.

So for me it was a mad rush to get home from work for a late lunch to see the breakfast going down and then an early rendezvous to see him a little more relaxed in his evening.

The weekends were more relaxed again as he was either Skyping by the pool or in a shopping centre explaining the differences between life there and here and the way things were done there.

As time went by it was becoming more and more challenging for me to see the pool scenario and I sometimes battled with the need to see him and the feeling I had drawn the wrong end of the stick. But sometimes showing love and care in a tangible way meant being creative.

With Steve away I embraced *Gourmet Traveller* magazine. One of my extended family had given the subscription for a gift and little did they know what they had done because each month I would rush to the postbox in hope of its arrival. I had morphed into a cookaholic.

Gone were the old school recipes of my past – in with the new and ever so special selection on offer month after month. Admittedly there were a number of disasters, but as time went by I put on my newly acquired apron and cooked myself silly. Many of my clients and family members benefited from this new development and even Steve was surprised when served poisson wrapped in prosciutto, stuffed with prunes, herbs and orange served with caramelised beans followed by spiced plum clafoutis and vanilla bean baked crème.

Without realising it at the time, I had found my mode of therapy, which not only put to rest others' concern that I was fading away but also gave me another method of cheering up others and bringing wide-eyed surprise to those I now sometimes entertained. Food and the wonder of it had somehow helped ease a level of pain.

It's a strange thing when your partner flies in and flies out. Every time was a build-up of both excitement and expectation, of preparation and an underlying hint of dread. I wanted to make it special for Steve and so I cooked his favourite things beforehand to save time when together – I didn't want to waste a single minute.

If it was a three-day turnaround, it was really tough. Steve would be exhausted but so glad to be home. Just to go for a leisurely walk outside in the fresh air was now a treat for him and he was starting to really appreciate the simple things that used to be just part of normal living. He was beginning to see our neighbourhood in a completely new light.

HOMECOMING

I would find myself looking at him a lot and observing him when I thought he didn't realise.

It was becoming strange to view Steve in this way and even after he had just arrived, I found myself starting to project how much longer we had until he was to leave.

It was such a tricky balance between just enjoying the moment for what it was and thinking ahead to how many hours were left until departure.

Sometimes emotions were so conflicted that I found I just had to keep busy by doing his washing, ironing shirts ready for the week ahead, or simply read a book while he sat at his computer in the lounge room. Just being in the same room was a precious thing.

And then before I knew it the day had come.

Farewell again. It was supposed to get easier.

I thought that by now I would have developed some better coping skills, but no, after he'd gone I would slowly roam around the rooms, having a little chat to myself about getting it together and getting a grip, reminding myself that we were fortunate in so many ways and that yes he would return, hopefully sooner rather than later.

Living apart had brought some important lessons for me. I realised how much I had depended on Steve for support. I missed his help in some of the everyday workings of life and my pain intensified as a result. Shopping was a major issue as

I couldn't carry any load, so it meant I needed to shop often and light and this of course used more energy and time.

I missed being physically fit. I missed being able to do what I wanted, when I wanted and I missed Steve. Sometimes a surprise can heal a whole range of hurt.

Anniversary

After years of marriage this anniversary was a significant one. Even after so long it still somehow seemed that time had passed like a blink of an eye; but if I were to scroll through the years, the shifts, the jobs, the plans, the mistakes, the achievements, the people, the travel, the family, the heartache and the joys, I would always reach the same conclusion.

Steve really was the love of my life and he was what gave purpose and meaning to all our hopes and dreams.

The last three-day visit hadn't been great, because Steve had been overly tired, frustrated with some areas of his work, and didn't really have enough time to relax before jetting off again. It was on this visit that I felt he had simply moved into another hotel, quite clearly the five stars he'd been experiencing of late had made an impression without him even realising.

I followed along after him, gathered up his dirty clothes, washed and pressed them, put the toilet seat down numerous times and basically put away anything he had used.

HOMECOMING

He was distant. Something had changed – some kind of shift had happened. This was new territory and I couldn't make sense of what had happened and whether I was somehow imagining it.

What a strange thing it is to love. What a conflicting emotion love is. In its fullness it can scale mountains, shift immovable objects, fill every crevice of the universe and leave you completely baffled at the same time.

I searched high and low, looked at all the angles, revisited the many conversations, asked light and breezy Skype questions and looked for any noticeable signs which could help me understand what was happening to Steve and where he had gone.

Fear started to work its way into the web that distance can weave. I had to tread carefully. I encouraged and listened and hoped that time would soon tell what was happening to my brave man.

It took a solid two weeks of Skyping to gradually work through the maze that was causing Steve's stress. Solitude for him had a *very* different meaning to what I experienced. I had always felt as time progressed that Steve's world had opened up and expanded with new challenges, new people, friends, places and stimulus. A place I was not part of.

My world had become the complete reverse. It had closed in, to a very small space. It was predictable because it revolved around pain and its constraints to my work and what could be managed, then required rest to start the next day all over again.

Even though Steve wasn't around, he knew exactly what my life was like, there were no surprises. It was consistent. It was no threat to him.

We were living polar opposite lives. A fundamental part of our relationship was based on honest open communication, trust and the innate knowledge that the other person was always on your side, ready to back you up or support you when the need arose. A team.

Sometimes it was confronting to battle to find a solution if someone was not behaving well, to search to the inner depths of yourself to understand and look honestly at poor behaviour or selfishness. To take a long hard look at yourself.

Usually these hard times had only built a greater strength and understanding. Usually there would be some common ground. Usually we would end up together, sometimes worn out, sometimes humbled.

But always together.

Steve broke down. It was the homemade biscuits that did it. It was his birthday and he was a long way from home. He had missed coming home for Christmas and I felt it would be completely unbearable for him to be alone for his birthday on top of that.

HOMECOMING

There had been no home visits for three months and Skyping was taking its toll as he was travelling a lot and often couldn't fit the time zones to connect.

So I cooked.

Ridiculous as it seems now, I spent hundreds of dollars posting a present of homemade biscuits and cookies to him every week before his birthday, so that week four culminated in his actual birthday present, which was a little tea pot and tea ... supposedly to go with the biscuits.

At last, the sheer absurdity of posting biscuits week in, week out to the other side of the world stripped aside the wall, opened up the gate and revealed just how hard Steve had been trying to protect me from his desperate loneliness and the conflicts inside he was struggling with.

He wanted to provide so that I didn't need to struggle on with work. He missed everything about home and didn't want to let me down by appearing weak.

We had been protecting each other and in doing so, had inadvertently built a barrier between ourselves. It was when Steve lifted to the camera a cellophane bag that we both broke down into tears of laughter and relief.

I had never considered that with air travel to hot humid places, my biscuits may not respond well to such intense changes of temperature. What I saw before me was a huge blob of a biscuit, the mother of all biscuits was being waved in the air. They had all melted together, given up their fight to be individual, succumbed to the intense heat while travelling to the other side of the world, formed a mess and then reset.

I watched Steve demolish the lot before my eyes and sighed. Ah, there he was, home at last.

The Market

It was Saturday and I was finishing with my last client when I received a brief text message from my niece. 'Are you planning to go to the market today? If so, we could meet there for coffee.'

Whether that was my plan or not I would always jump at the chance of seeing my niece Sally and her husband Michael, because they were two of my favourite people in the world and I would work around any plans to make it happen. This was exciting, I loved their company and the coffee was fantastic at the market. They knew where to meet.

So I went about my business, slowly cleaned up work after finishing with the last client, went home, changed and started walking to the market. The day was sunny with some cloud, though this as I knew didn't mean anything in particular. November could still be unpredictable so I took a small umbrella just in case and a bag to buy a few odds and ends.

I did a lap of the market and was just turning around the corner to the coffee place which was situated in an internal walkway when I stopped dead in my tracks. I caught my breath and stood with my mouth open. Stunned. There they were. All three of them.

In a dream film scenario I would drop what I was holding, burst into tears, run over to them and throw my arms around Steve. He would lift me off the ground and swing me in the air amid laughter and the surprise of those around us.

Instead, I slowly made my way towards them and managed a gentle, tentative hug for Steve. My face must have been hilarious because they were all in fits of laughter. I was in complete shock. Then their words filled my ears as they divulged the story, all interrupting each other in waves of excitement and arm movements.

Tears ran down my cheeks as I heard the surprise had been planned for the anniversary when Steve found he was nearby for work … in Singapore … he was so close he couldn't pass up the opportunity. Eight hours away didn't seem all that close to me, but I didn't care, I was grinning from one face to the next as I heard that Sally and Michael had picked him up from the airport, had breakfast together and then brought him over to Prahran to rendezvous at the market.

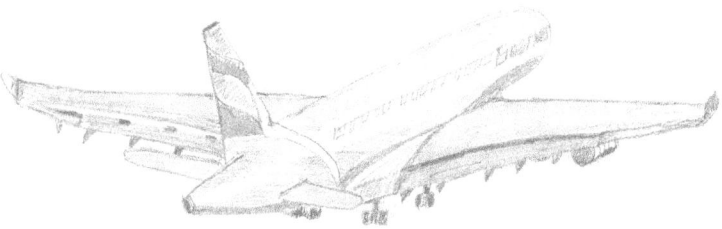

A CURRAWONG SOMERSAULT

He had one day and was to fly back the next day. This was the best gift anyone had *ever* given me. This meant the world. With this one enormous effort Steve had just shown me what I was worth. Nothing else now mattered.

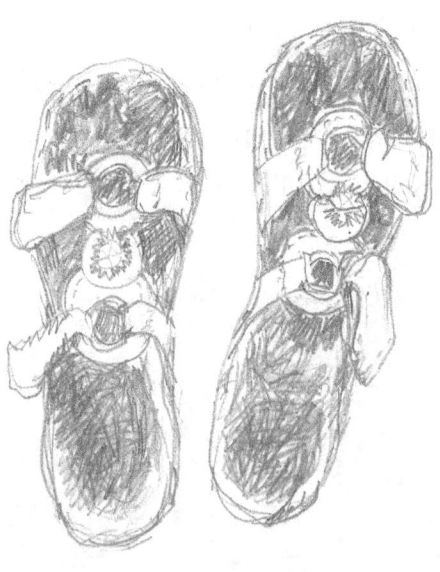

SUMMER 2019

CHAPTER 11

Summer 2019

The sun was streaming into the bedroom through the timber venetian blinds as if they weren't even there. It was to be another hot day ahead and it wasn't even 7 am. Nights like this cause mayhem on the roads and a strange unhinged atmosphere in the streets.

It's a cocktail no one wants to drink, but those who don't have the comfort of air-conditioning have to do the best they can, they appear dishevelled and bleary-eyed with something not quite in place.

The tie is a little crooked, the collar on one side not sitting flat, the skirt zip is just off centre and the make-up is at its bare minimum. After five nights over 40 degrees, weather had now superseded coffee as the major topic of conversation for Melbournians. Surviving the heat now binds us together.

New records reached in heatwave. Melbourne airport recorded Melbourne's hottest temperature this summer at 46 degrees on the 25th of January 2019.

News had it covered completely.

We all watched pictures of sweltering streets, limp bodies fanning themselves, slumped under trees, dogs being carried for their walks in the evening, overheated cars waiting for assistance, someone showed they could *fry an egg* on the bonnet of their sedan.

This was in contrast to kids running under hoses, jumping into anything that vaguely looked like water, people sitting in fountains in parks, standing baking in the sun at the beach and others lying in a bath of ice water.

Whatever angle the media took, it either made me feel 100 times hotter or at the very least brought a smile to my face. Things would surely change soon.

Thankfully my work had air-conditioning and clients would arrive already very red in the face and gradually come back to life before my eyes, then as the session progressed, gradually the red face was back in position ready for their departure. Many showers were had at my business over this period and everyone benefited from the ability to still exercise and not kill themselves trying to do the same type of thing outside.

It never ceased to amaze me how many people still tried to exercise outside in extreme heat. No matter the warnings, the media, the doctor's advice, there were still those that gave extra work to the ambulance and emergency services. Heat exhaustion can be deadly even without exercise. Most of my clients were H_2O challenged at the best of times, so it was a constant struggle to find new and creative ways to get the liquid into them. One 80-year-old male client who has a wicked sense of humour and sings the theme song to his football club whenever possible announces, 'I come to training to get my two glasses of water for the week.'

On day two of 'the wave' as everyone was now calling it, Steve had a profound idea. This was not uncommon, but considering the extreme weather it was pretty impressive.

'Why don't we bunk up at your studio on the floor? At least there is air-conditioning there and we'll get some sleep? It can be like camping!'

Brilliance at its best. Both Steve and I loved camping. At least we did about 20 years ago and it still held the misty aura of freedom, open space, getting down to basics and bucking the norm. Perfect. So it was decided. We packed our overnight bags, pillows and light cotton blanket and drove over to the studio. Piling all the rubber mats on top of each other gave the basis of a bed and then it was the huge decision of exactly where to position ourselves.

Steve was very keen to be directly underneath the air-conditioner and so in the interest of happiness and a quick decision, I agreed. Thankfully it was Saturday night so we didn't need to be up early the next day for work, so after a lovely cold glass of water along with the chilled bottle of white wine we'd purchased on the way we hit the sack.

One thing was absolutely sure. It was cold. It was *really* cold and my teeth were chattering as I clutched the cotton blanket around my neck. I listened to the snoring beside me and observed half a body on the mat and half on the floor.

Amazing.

I carefully got up and altered the temperature gauge to non blast and proceeded to wander around the small studio to sort out the crick in my neck and one hip that didn't like the idea of camping.

It had been 10 years since I had started business there. I loved this space. It was small but I knew it was better to have a small lovely space rather than a cavernous dump.

Both Steve and I had often run our own businesses over the years. Some worked well, others were best forgotten, but we had given it a go and worked hard to try and get ahead. It was easier said than done beacuse working this way meant there were no paid holidays or sick leave and every dollar had to be accounted for to make ends meet and cover business costs.

I ran my finger over the sliding door handle. Even after all this time I found joy in sliding the huge black gloss double door that separated the main working space to another room, previously used as a bedroom. The door slides across to form a wall barrier between the main area and the bedroom now converted to stretch and flexibility. Floor-to-ceiling windows flood light into all three sides creating a glowing inviting space. The theme is soft grey and white and the only real contrast as such is a hint of my favourite colour here and there in artwork or a random chair.

I smiled as I remember my first viewing of the property. At that stage it was being rented out as an apartment but had been on the market for some time. I had to move out of where I was currently renting because the owner wanted to take possession so I had to act quickly to find an alternative place to operate from. On arrival, the agent greeted me at the footpath, which I immediately thought was very impressive.

It was always so nice to be surprised by extra care or service and this was something I myself always hoped was appreciated by my clients, but often seemed to be quite rare, especially when dealing with real estate rentals or sales departments.

It was an upstairs apartment with dual licencing, so it could be converted to a business situation if required. Everything

I had seen to date had been way too expensive and had either needed major renovations to put in a bathroom and security or the standard of fit out just didn't feel right. I also needed adequate parking for clients and easy access for those who were more challenged physically.

All the way up the stairs the agent talked through the positives. As he stood at the door entry he paused, looked me in the eye and said, 'Just look beyond what you see and you'll see the potential'.

The first thing that hit me was the smell. Stale. Smoky and a strange waft that made me screw up my nose and reach for a tissue. Next were the flies and one had just tried to fly directly up my nose. I spluttered and coughed. All the while the agent smiled and coaxed, reassured and led. He was in a class of his own. It was nearing month-end so perhaps the budget deadlines were putting on the pressure?

Whatever it was he glossed over the yellow walls, the red wine stains on the carpet and furniture, the pizza boxes stacked all over the table and the bong-making facilities sitting comfortably in the mess, the clothing thrown all over the floor in the bedroom and the blinds hanging at odd angles next to each other.

I had no idea how long I had been inside, but I knew I had to get out of there as quickly as possible or I would throw up. I put a hand up to the agent to ask him to stop for a second and let me take stock. He obliged, as he too needed to wipe his nose. I took out my phone and took photos of each of the rooms. I wrote down the obvious things that needed doing and then noted the pluses.

I asked him to send me through the dimensions, the cost details and outgoings, and in minutes I was out of there. Fresh air at last. This was to be my new place of business.

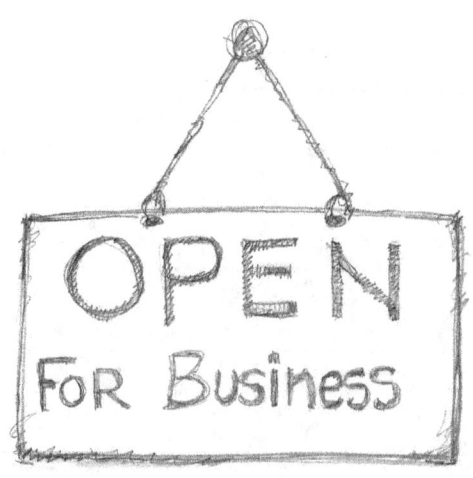

CHAPTER 12

Trusting Your Gut

Intuition? Who really knows. A sixth sense? Maybe. Coincidence? Possible.

Many things had happened in my life over the years that have given me a sense that there is more going on that meets the eye.

When lying in bed awake with something going on other than pain and discomfort, I found a sense of calm in systematically going back through history adding up all the times that important things had happened. All the things that amazed and baffled me at the same time were lined up like prizes, remembered and appreciated, polished and admired.

Some were small and seemingly inconsequential and others were major life events, where I had learnt important lessons. Many and varied, big and small. There were many – so many in fact that often I would find myself nodding off when only halfway through the memorised list. But even as my eyes finally closed to sleep I'd smile in satisfaction and gratitude, knowing that these gifts had been given for some unknown reason and I held them dear. Careful never, never to take them for granted.

No one spoke about things much when I was a child. It was my place to just go with the flow, do what I was told and do the best I could in the limitations that were being the youngest. I knew what was expected of me and enjoyed the freedom that my brothers had never experienced because they had worn them down by the time I'd arrived as a somewhat unexpected surprise.

It was unusual to have a child so late in life and my parents had to take many precautions.

My mother had to rest a lot in the early stages of pregnancy and was given numerous drugs to assist with the complications that arose on the way. This alone was probably enough to create tension in the household, but as time progressed my brothers made a firm pact that they would have to stick together now that there was to be another mouth to feed.

They had already done the hard yards and the last thing they needed was a disruption to the system now working so well.

Little did they realise that they would be landed with a little sister and this little girl wanted for all her worth to be like her brothers, to do what they did and be loved by them.

I was always referred to as 'your sister' and often when our mother was unwell it fell on my brothers to take care of me and keep me out of harm's way. Somehow I survived.

For the most part my brothers allowed me to tag along, but many times I was left behind, unable to remember how to find my way home. Regardless, I learnt that sometimes it was fun to play with them and other times it certainly was not. I learnt to amuse myself.

I loved to run. I loved athletics and anything that involved movement and dance. My parents recognised this after my early years religiously spent dancing and performing on the front nature strip to anyone going by and perhaps it was the embarrassment of this or the sheer wearing down of my enthusiasm that determined my destiny for ballet classes. I will always remember the joy of my first outfit. This was the first time in my life that I had clothes that were my very own.

A day of extreme nervousness and excitement mixed together like a frothy strawberry milkshake, and this was almost too much to bear for a young six-year-old.

It was the softness of the little pink ballet shoes that captured my heart and the smell was like nothing else. I was so excited I secretly wore them to bed each night for a week before my mother noticed one morning and suggested it wasn't such a good idea long term.

Even when I stopped the night routine, I'd still try them on whenever I was by myself in my room and point my toes in the positions I was learning, marvelling at their beauty and more importantly how they made me feel. Special.

I was the youngest in my class and was thrilled when the local newspaper photographer came and took a photo of me *in position* inside the old church hall where we rehearsed. The sunshine beamed through the stained-glass window lighting me up just at the right moment.

This was my very first official event and everyone in the family thought it was fairly special.

Truth be known, if the sport was finished for the week and there are no new births to photograph then a newspaper reporter can get very desperate. Very desperate indeed.

Having been born to older parents I somehow always felt that they were old.

My mother would always need an afternoon rest and she would often lie down with me chattering or singing next to her. My father was often away for weeks with his work commitments and so the boys were left to their own devices after school and I just fitted in with whatever was scheduled for the day.

There was a rhythm of sorts. Time passed.

TRUSTING YOUR GUT

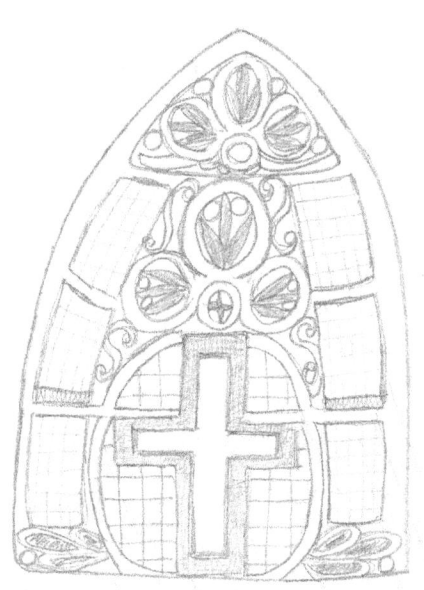

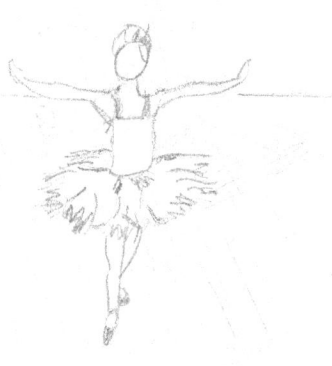

The boys were both enrolled in Cubs and then Scouts because they were getting up to mischief together and it was decided that these activities would solve a lot of those issues.

Once every few years the Scout Association organised a Jubilee. It was an event where all troops around Australia converged at a large site to meet and showcase the many skills that both Cubs and Scouts of all ages had learnt, culminating at the end with a massive celebration and bonfire where each troop would be rewarded with a new badge.

Very exciting, especially for a country town.

Many visiting families required accommodation and so our family offered the small caravan housed in our backyard next to the garage.

Small is the understatement. It was shaped like a half moon on wheels and as kids we would often play inside it and pretend it was a shop or whatever came to mind.

Our holidays were predictable. It was the caravan, the annexe, the Holden packed to the brim and a road trip to somewhere in a three-hour radius.

A scouting family had accepted the offer of the caravan and they were to stay for a week.

This had never happened before. They were a family of four with two boys of similar ages to my brothers and they would be sharing our facilities and most meals.

It was a game changer for me.

Derek, the oldest of the boys, had taken an instant shine to me and treated me with such kindness that I almost didn't know how to respond. He had evidently always wanted a sister and so thought he'd like to adopt me, at least while they were with us. I was instantly shy and didn't know how to be anymore, but over the course of the week he gained my trust and by day five we were playing monopoly and making up plays and performing them. He wrote a lovely message in my autograph book and I was beginning to wonder if perhaps I could go and live with Derek and his family. I had made my first true friend, and he was a boy. The world had shifted and changed.

The day had come and they were leaving. I was devastated and couldn't bring myself to go to the front gate to wave them goodbye so instead I lay on my bed clutching the autograph book wondering whether he really would write to me as he said he would. Would I ever survive this feeling of loss? I stayed there all day contemplating the options.

Sadly by now Mrs Ubergang's cat had passed away so I had no other point of reference and could not discuss the issue with anyone else.

I'd have to figure it out on my own.

A week had passed and no letter had been received. Time was dragging and nothing seemed to take my interest, even ballet was an effort and that was not usual.

I noticed the quiet around the dinner table. The chewing was the same, the clock ticked just the same, everyone was seated in their normal positions, a word was said here and there, but there was a definite change – more quiet than the normal quiet.

My mother tried to start conversations by asking questions but the answers were short and before long it was back to the ticking clock.

Everyone missed the family who stayed, what a gap they had made. It was almost too much to bear.

It was Sunday and it was nearly time to go over to Nanna and Grandad's for lunch. I'd changed out of my good clothes and was ready before anyone else so went out into the backyard to wander around the woodheap and back fence that housed my father's shed. I loved it around the back.

The smell of the wood and the neighbour's trees that hung over the fence where sometimes the light would filter through the wooden palings and I could see their veggie garden or watch the kids play on their swing. It squeaked whenever it went up so I always knew when they were outside and sometimes we would throw a ball over the fence to each other if it was too late to go around and play. It was a special place.

Not for anyone else, but I loved the colour of the ground here, the wood, the smells, the old axe wedged into the largest woodblock, the insects that darted around in the air when the sun was setting and the way it made me feel. If I sat very still a bird would come and sit on the fence. It didn't seem to mind me being there, so I'd sit and watch. Sit and listen. Sit and wait for the next thing to happen.

I went to the rear of the woodheap and looked around. Things had been moved around a bit and we certainly hadn't needed a fire in summer, so I was curious as to why the wood stack had been disturbed. Quite clearly it had been stacked to make a kind of step up to the rear fence.

Someone has been busy, I thought, *but why?* It looked like an escape route. Maybe the boys had been playing around when Derek was here?

Maybe they went over to the neighbours place? The kids behind were much younger so I couldn't make sense of that. My brothers would never be seen dead playing with anyone younger than themselves and even if Derek had encouraged them, they wouldn't get sucked into doing that. No way.

With more purpose, I looked around further in the hope of a clue, and then my name was called. Time was running out. Then I saw them. Tucked between two bits of wood were a pair of thongs. Not ordinary thongs. These were the Indian variety that were made of leather and had a woven toe hole for the biggest toe to slip into. They were thin and almost too delicate to touch. Brown and I just knew they would smell divine. These thongs had been on my wish list for a couple of years.

All my friends at school had them and wore them with their Levi jeans and cheesecloth tops. I would never ask my mother for such an extravagance as I knew we had to be careful to make ends meet. We never went hungry and didn't miss what we didn't have, but sometimes it was difficult being the odd one out when it came down to the latest fashion accessory that many of my girlfriends enjoyed.

I quickly looked around, stepped onto the couple of wobbly blocks in front and balanced precariously until the thongs were in my grasp. Retracing my steps I jumped back onto the ground and dusted them off. What on earth? This had to be one of the weirdest things to happen in a while. Whose could they be? And what were they doing in the woodheap?

I knew at once. I took off my shoes and socks and held my breath.

They were an exact fit. Someone had heard my wish. I laughed out loud, jumped up and down on the spot and cried, 'Thank you ... thank you so very much!'

This was a gift I would treasure forever. I never told anyone this story, as it sounded kind of strange and silly when said out loud. So I just told my parents I'd found them in the woodheap and they were happy with that explanation.

It was only a few months after that the neighbours at the back reported that their home had been broken into and we should all keep our wits about us.

TRUSTING YOUR GUT

A CURRAWONG SOMERSAULT

CHAPTER 13

A Getaway October 2019

As a child, I didn't make friends easily. In many ways I was shy, which seems in strange contrast to skipping around the front nature strip in petticoats. Perhaps the other girls didn't understand the joy of running freely in pasture or jumping off the bridge into the irrigation channel. Whatever the reasons I was more comfortable with boys, so making a true girlfriend was something I really treasured.

I sat opposite my friend Megan and observed. This was the second week I had noticed that she wasn't her usual self. She chatted as per usual, smiled between sips of ice coffee and then found her phone to show a text message and photo she needed to share, she then looked around, sighed and excused herself. Nature called, so I took this opportunity to reposition myself. This was one of the many cafés I knew in our area that had high stools that I could stand and lean against. Sitting was still painful and managing in this way meant that I could show some semblance of normality, without screaming in pain. Megan and I often met like this. Somehow the world axis would shift off centre, and cause unimaginable mayhem in the universe, if we didn't see each other at least once a week.

It was law and we were law-abiding citizens.

We had fallen nicely into catching up at a nearby café after Megan's weekly exercise session, something that Megan thought was hilarious, considering the size of the ice cream scoop she was now stirring in her glass.

Megan returned. I needed to be careful. Megan had endured a great deal of stress lately and the signs were beginning to show. We knew each other very well, and I realised that Megan had probably already guessed that I was onto her. We were blessed with a unique relationship because not only did we share the same sense of humour, but we had created an unusual language that made complete sense to us and often left others perplexed. A subtle change to a word, an emphasis or melodic lilt to a sentence, sometimes a look was enough. Our friendship had evolved to the extend that we had our own special way to communicate.

A GETAWAY OCTOBER 2019

I let out a sigh, to match the latest one that had escaped Megan unknowingly. There was a pause.

'So I was just thinking … can you remember the last time we went away for a weekend together? Seems like years to me … any thoughts?'

Megan tilted her head and a slight smile tried not to appear. 'Oh definitely years I'd reckon … my memory may be getting worse … but at a guess … it would have to be at least ten, why?'

I nodded and began to rustle around in my bag. Tissues, icepacks, medication, sunglasses, paper and pen, diary, reading glasses, it was a great feat of discovery when I found my phone. I scrolled through my photos, looked at my friend, passed her the phone and watched her face.

'Does your memory recollect this?'

Megan also rummaged around in her bag and found her glasses. My how things had changed. It now seemed that between the pair of us, we were constantly either looking for something, or trying to remember something or a combination of both.

The laugh that exploded from Megan startled the waitress who was passing behind her.

The poor young girl nearly dropped the tray full of drinks she was carrying, so Megan swiftly apologised and then turned and made a face at me. 'That was *your* fault you know … how embarrassment, that could have been a major disaster

… what were you thinking? … That last mouthful went directly up my nose!' There she was, this was Megan at her finest. There were so many things that I loved about my dear friend, but one thing which sat very high on the list was her wonderful sense of humour.

We shared the same one, in fact we had often amused ourselves for hours when driving to gigs, simply by making up things along the way. The more tired, the more ridiculous routines and songs became. It was the absurdity we enjoyed. Pity any poor soul who had to endure our repartee for any length of time.

It was a strange gift. Many times over the years, other people would find themselves unwittingly joining in. They'd throw in a line or just laugh along at the right time. It was ad lib and completely unrehearsed. We poked fun, exaggerated everything, and changed words to songs, often to the point of no return.

My laugh echoed. 'Oh it's *my* fault now is it? And just who was snorting up the coffee? You nearly scared the poor girl to death, in fact you were almost wearing a lovely shade of pink cider … perfect match with your gym gear … me thinks.'

Megan huffed, determined not to laugh again. Allowing my friend time to recover, I promptly changed the subject. 'Oh I don't know … I'm missing wearing a hat … and it's been so long since I've been stuck in traffic looking at roadworks ... that it seems only the sensible thing to do ...

I'm in need of an adventure ... it's been too long ... and I've completely forgotten how to pack a bag. Are you coming, or not?'

Megan now had her mouth open, so I waited. This was not a good look and sometimes it was hard to read the signs. Megan sighed. Thankfully it was a different sigh to all the previous, as this one had a slight smirk attached to it.

Warburton Ranges October 2019

Megan loaded the suitcase, pillow, cooler bag, another bag and numerous other bits and pieces, into the boot of her car. 'For crying out loud, how long are you intending to stay? I thought it was just the weekend ... are you on for a month or something?'

Pursing my lips I exclaimed, 'Oh how unkind ... [said in my most posh voice] ... as you well know. I am completely out of practice and therefore had no choice but to bring everything I own, just in case!'

Megan laughed. It was good to hear her laugh. 'Well it appears we will not be going hungry. There's enough food here to feed a small village.'

Without hesitation the reply, 'Well then, just as well we are going to a small village ... Warby only has about two thousand residents doesn't it? So that will be absolutely perfect, everyone shall be suitably fed.'

After arranging the pillow underneath me, readjusting icepacks to hit the exact target, putting on the travelling cap and taking a sip of water, I smiled at my friend. This may well kill me physically, but all the other benefits would be off the scale and well worth it.

Stevie Wonder was accompanying our journey and I knew that was a good omen. It was about 76 kilometres to Warburton and the small township nestled comfortably in the Yarra Valley, there was a pub, a bakery, with the best meat pies known to man, a couple of restaurants, and an eclectic mix of shops which specialised in spells and mystic remedies.

We may explore them, we may not. It would depend how things evolved. This was another thing I loved about Megan: she was often happy to simply go with the flow.

We had stopped a couple of times, so that I could stretch my legs and Stevie had disembarked at the last stop, which was good, because that then allowed space for Nat King Cole and his daughter Natalie to travel comfortably with us.

I hoped they didn't mind that we embellished their songs. Megan thought they were being polite. 'I just don't understand why they continuously get the words wrong to their own songs!' We laughed at ourselves and how very amusing we were.

A GETAWAY OCTOBER 2019

Singing along to songs passed the time as I watched two nurseries and a rose garden specialist go by.

It seemed that nature was a major highlight in this area, and I couldn't believe my eyes when we drove past a lotus farm and gasped with delight.

I absolutely loved waterlilies and lotus plants the flowers are so beautiful, and even the tall seed pods are a work of art, in their own right. It was closed, so I settled back in my seat, ever so slightly disappointed.

A few kilometres down the road something strange happened. I was gazing out the window looking at the passing fields, when a very clear thought presented itself. I found myself viewing a lush green garden, with walkways either side of a dense hedge of rosemary. I peeked over the hedge and what did I see? Tucked among the foliage was a deep, white enamel bath, filled to the brim with water.

A nearby maple tree gently embraced it and the orange and yellow leaves were set alight by a filtered ray of light. The colour was superb, but what I saw next took my breath away. Nestled in the bath were waterlilies in various colours, and rising above them stood huge lotus flowers, proud and erect. Deep, deep pink blooms. Some were open and some were closed. I smiled as I saw a little wren fly to the rim of the bath and take a sip. I blinked, and blinked again, and just as quickly as it had arrived, the image was gone. I looked across at Megan.

A CURRAWONG SOMERSAULT

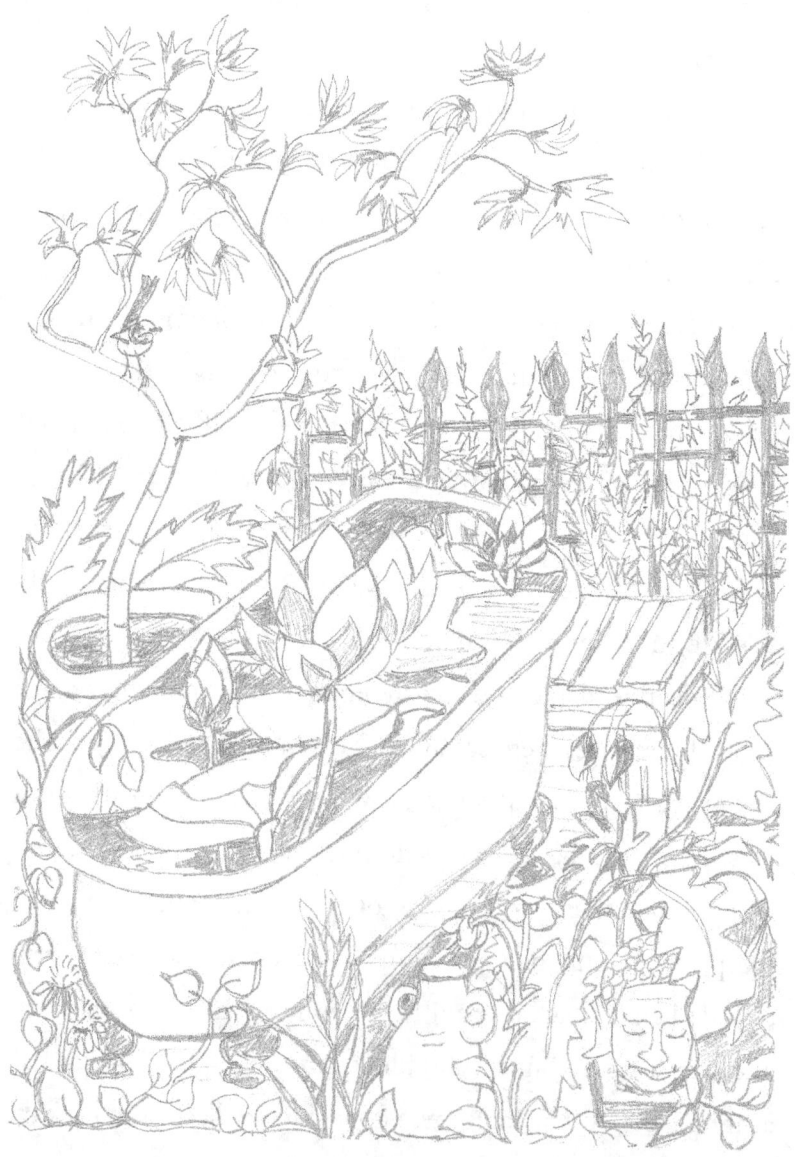

Well, that was interesting, perhaps I wasn't used to such fresh, clean mountain air?

As if on cue, the mountains suddenly appeared and it was so beautiful to see them rising majestically to greet the sky. The cloud was quite low around the peaks, and a blue haze turned them from grey to deep green. Simultaneously and quite surprisingly, we both began to yawn. 'Oh excuse me for keeping you awake young lady. I didn't realise that the conversation had deteriorated to that degree.'

I laughed. 'Oh pardon me [as I stifled another] but who was just yawning at the same time?'

There was nothing we could both do but laugh, because something strange had just happened. We yawned our way into Warburton and eventually gave up trying to stop ourselves.

Something was letting go and we allowed it to happen.

The wooden balcony completely took up the front view of the cottage. It stood high against the hill, and it was quite clear, even when driving up the steep drive, that the view from above would be absolutely breathtaking. We drove under the carport, and the next thing that I saw made me clap my hands together like an excited child. 'A fire, a fire. Oh Megan how divine, there' a fire!'

'Well ... yes ... that was part of the surprise ... who's a lucky girl then? It's probably been too long since your last good poke.' Megan laughed, enjoying her own joke. I huffed and had nothing to say to that one. We'd had lunch on the way, so once unpacked, we settled ourselves on the three-seater lounges, around a roaring fire. It was easy, Megan read her book while I foraged around outside for anything I could burn. We shared some wine while nibbling on a wonderful cheese platter that Megan had provided, and then I commenced dinner.

Chicken and mushroom pie, scalloped potatoes and whole beans, followed by an Italian celebration cake and raspberries. This was a celebration after all.

Megan politely left half her cake. 'I'm so full, I couldn't fit in a caraway seed.' She was used to eating small portions and this was a lot in one sitting. 'I will probably toss and turn all night as a result.' She smiled at me, I knew that look. She was happy and didn't care if she did.

We talked and didn't talk, read our books and went for walks, dozed, were silent, ventured out to explore the famous bakery to sample the award-winning pies and I poked the fire to my hearts content. A flock of five lorikeets swooped into a nearby tree, their tweets filling the air with an excitement that heralded a healthy meal was on offer. We gazed across the horizon.

The balcony didn't disappoint. The mountains folded into themselves, revealing brilliant flashes of coloured leaves as the sun shone through the moving clouds. It was brisk and the air was cold as it hit our lungs. Smoke wafted from nearby chimneys and I was called to start our own fire.

Chicken and Mushroom Pie

Ingredients:

1 kg diced chicken thigh

½ kg chicken mince

6-8 cocktail potatoes, cut in half

1 large brown onion, finely chopped

2-3 garlic cloves finely chopped

8-12 Swiss mushrooms halved

1 heaped teaspoon seeded mustard

1 teaspoon honey

Rind and juice of 1 lemon

Chopped parsley and coriander, some fresh thyme

½ cup cream and a little plain flour

A splash of Worcestershire sauce, or light soy sauce

A squirt of tomato sauce

Sea salt and pepper to taste

Puff pastry sheets and egg to glaze

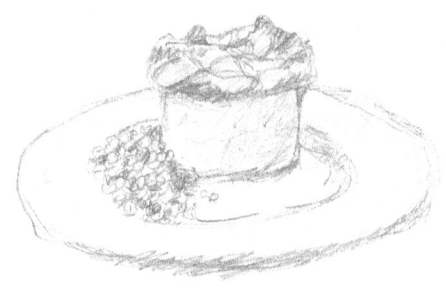

Method:

Preheat moderate oven to 180ºC (160ºC fan forced).

Prepare onion, garlic, mushrooms and wash herbs.

In a non-stick pan, with a little oil, cook the diced chicken thigh in batches until slightly brown. Remove and place on absorbent paper. Once complete, set aside in a large bowl.

In the same pan, brown and gently cook the chicken mince, pressing it with your spoon to ensure there are no clumps and it covers the pan evenly.

Once cooked, transfer to the large bowl of chicken pieces. Using the same pan, add a little oil and gently fry the onion and garlic with the teaspoon of honey until caramelised.

Transfer to bowl.

In a medium size saucepan, cook the potatoes until firm.

Meanwhile, gently pan fry the mushrooms with a little oil until just soft. Do not include all the liquid to the pie mix, if there is a lot. Drain potatoes and add to the large bowl.

Defrost the puff pastry sheets.

Mix all ingredients in the large bowl and add the seeded mustard, herbs, lemon zest and juice, cream, Worcestershire sauce, tomato sauce, salt and pepper.

Add a little plain flour, or corn flour. The amount will depend on how wet the mixture is. Try a heaped tablespoon first and see how it appears.

Grease a heavy cooking dish and spoon in the mixture. Alternatively use small ceramic dishes for individual pies.

Cut the pastry so it overlaps the sides and pinch around the edges. Pierce the top of the pastry to allow the steam to escape, and egg wash the pastry.

Cook for 30-40 minutes until the pastry is golden and fluffed. Serve with steamed beans.

Scalloped Potatoes

Ingredients:
6-8 large Desiree potatoes
1 garlic clove, finely diced
Sea salt and pepper (white pepper is preferred)
½ cup cream
½ cup milk
A little butter
A sprinkle of pimenton (smoked paprika)
Finely grated parmesan cheese

Method:
Preheat moderate oven 180ºC (160ºC fan forced).

Peel the potatoes, wash them and let them sit in a bowl of water for a few minutes to remove some of the starch.

Rub the bottom of a ceramic dish with butter.

Dice the garlic and sprinkle on the bottom of the dish.

Dry the potatoes and slice as finely as possible.

Layer the slices in the dish, starting at and edge and working down towards you, overlapping as you go, until the bottom of the dish is covered. Sprinkle a little salt and pepper and complete another layer of potato.

Salt and pepper again and add another layer. Continue until the dish is full, leaving about an inch gap at the top, to allow for juices.

Once full, add milk and dollop the cream over the top.

Cover the dish with grated cheese, sprinkle with paprika, and add a couple of knobs of butter.

Cook 40 minutes until golden (wise to put dishes on a baking tray to capture any spillage).

Italian Celebration Cake (Migliaccio Napoletano)
Ingredients:
1 litre full cream milk

125 g fine semolina

50 g unsalted butter, coarsely chopped

1 vanilla bean, seeds scraped

350 g ricotta

1 lemon, finely grated rind

5 eggs

350 g caster sugar

Pinch of sea salt

Pure icing sugar, for dusting

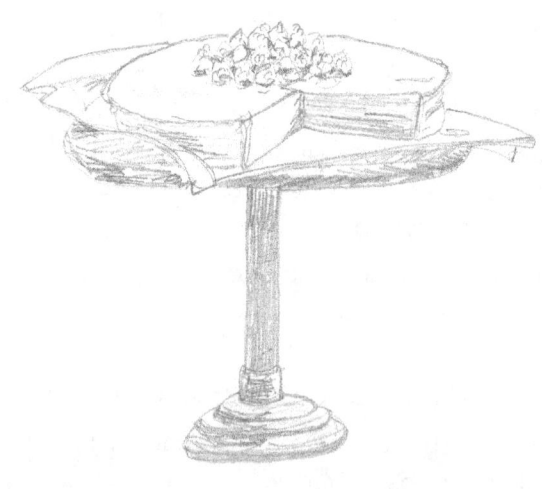

Method:

Preheat oven to 190°C (170°C fan forced).

Bring milk, semolina, butter, vanilla bean seeds and a pinch of sea salt just to the boil in a saucepan over medium heat.

Stir continuously (4-6 minutes) then place in a sink of cold water to cool, stirring frequently to stop skin forming (20-30 minutes).

Whisk ricotta and lemon rind in a medium bowl until a smooth cream and set aside.

In another large bowl, whisk eggs and sugar until just combined, then add ricotta mixture and whisk to combine. Don't overwork.

Make sure the semolina mixture is cool enough to add and then whisk until smooth.

Generously butter a 25 cm diameter, 5 cm deep cake tin (spring lock is best), and line the base with baking paper.

Pour in the batter, smooth the top and bake until the top is golden (50-60 minutes).

A good idea to move the cake, changing sides, halfway through if your oven heats unevenly.

Cool to room temperature in the tin, then turn out, or serve in the tin.

Cover the centre with fresh raspberries and fresh mint.

Dust with icing sugar.

It always tastes better the next day, if there's any left.

A CURRAWONG SOMERSAULT

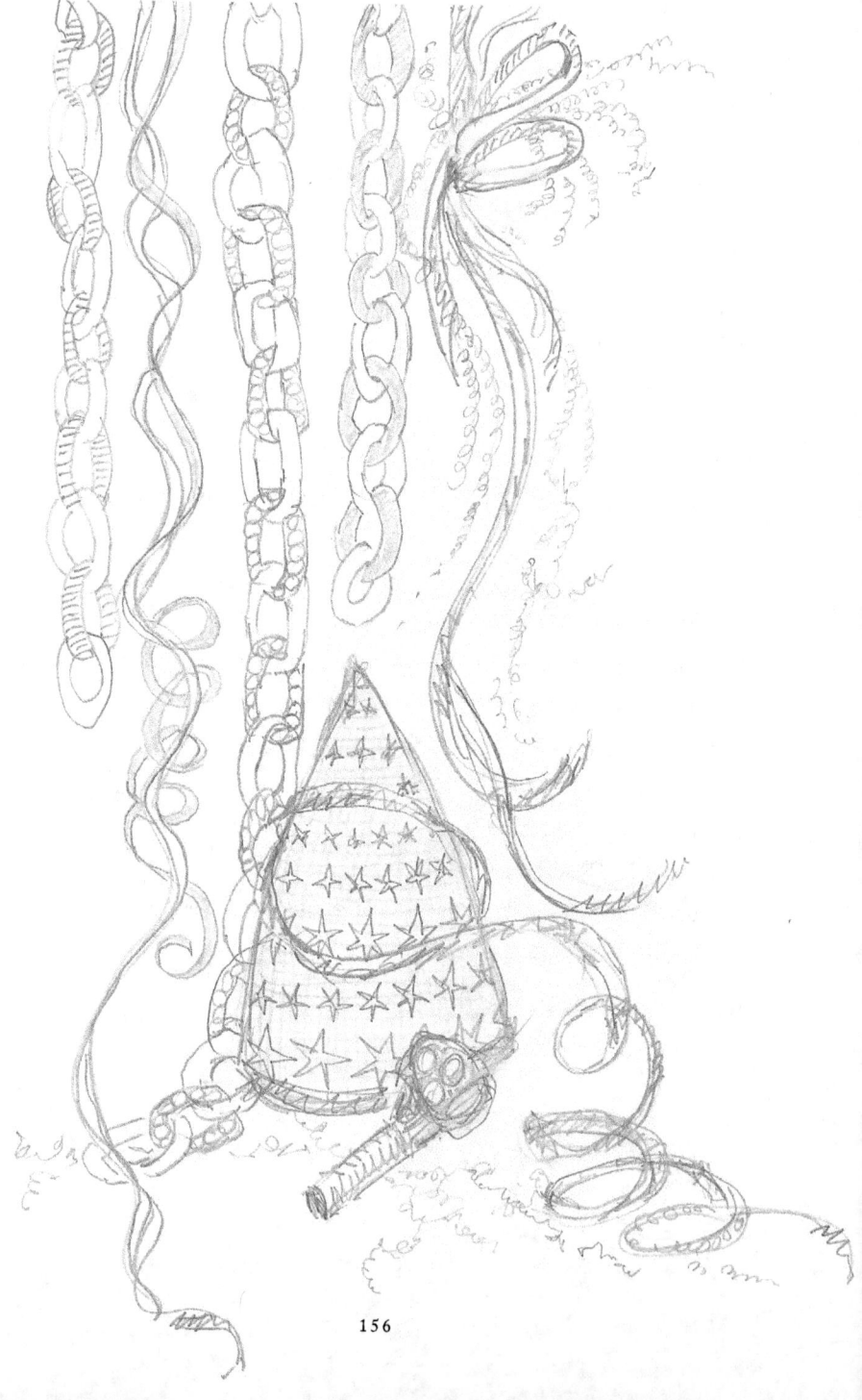

CHAPTER 14

A New Year 2020

A new year always filled me with a fresh sense of hope; 2020 sounded melodic, like a musical beat to my ears, and had a certain roll and lilt to it which added to the positivity.

I was optimistic and hopeful that my pain would disappear. Unrealistic expectations are rarely rewarded and I could now laugh at myself.

The pain clinic had taught me a great deal about prioritising and keeping things in perspective. Having more tools at my disposal meant I could pace myself, manage the pain and with Steve back at home, my life was once again complete.

It was the Year of the Rat and like all good Chinese symbols offered an explanation of what may lie ahead. The Rat was known to be resourceful, inquisitive and shrewd and it was to be a year of renewal and wealth. At last an improvement was on the way.

Christmas was always a chaotic and enjoyable time for us and our family.

It never ceased to amaze me how absolutely everybody we knew or vaguely knew all wanted to catch up and get together prior to Christmas and New Year, it was as if there would never be another opportunity. This happened each passing year, and so I had started organising little dinners and get-togethers weeks beforehand to try and ease the weariness that accumulated as everyone rushed to the finish line.

Most of my clients took a reasonable break over the Christmas period, as many of them were retired and had the means to travel or enjoy their holiday homes over the summer months, so I'd learnt to be careful throughout the year to cover the ongoing business costs while taking a forced break.

The buzz of the city was always exciting. I loved taking the tram into town to gaze at the Myer Christmas windows and stores stacked full of bright coloured boxes and decorations. The city always delivers a wonderful festive feel with lights and foliage decking the streets and shop fronts. The narrow laneways are a highlight of our Melbourne city centre and

A NEW YEAR 2020

provide not only an enormous variety of specialty shops but also some of the best street art in the world. The Block Arcade, with its beautiful mosaic floor and glass ceiling, houses the Hopetoun Tea Rooms, a glorious shop which has been receiving queues of visitors from around the globe since 1892. I would always find my way to the mall via this arcade, as the displays of cakes, slices, scones and delicate sandwiches were such a treat to the eye.

The Myer department store, located in the city mall, is renowned for its spectacular window display and each year they would choose a theme and then section off the area so that families and children of all ages could parade past and admire the wonder of it all.

This year it was gumnut babies in gumnut land, a magical interpretation of families of gumnuts all going about their business, making things for Christmas and celebrating life in the way gumnut babies do. I opted to shop instead of stop, as crowds were building up and my shopping endurance was somewhat limited due to pain thresholds.

For years I had missed this journey into the city, until I realised I needed to think about it differently. Even though I no longer had the luxury of taking my time to wander around the arcades and shops for hours, it dawned on me that finding another way would be worth a shot. What's the worst that could happen?

Pain would bite hard if I overdid movement and caused my hips to seize so that I hobbled around like an old woman. I couldn't concentrate and would need to retreat from everyone. I wouldn't be able to go to work and I'd be in bed for a couple of days … I knew the consequences … but I gave it a go.

The train runs direct to the city and I can stand. Tick. I'd travel light so I didn't load up my back. Tick. I'd choose only two to three shops to visit. Tick. And then the best of all, I would go to the Gallery at the Arts precinct and recover by lying on the floor like others did, and look up at the stained glass. Tick. Why hadn't I thought of this before? If ever pain went over my normal coping threshold the best thing I could do was to lie down. Not being able to sit comfortably meant that I was usually standing or lying down. My body recognised this as a recovery position and with deep-breathing techniques I'd learnt to find a way to stabilise pain and regroup.

The Gallery dedicated a whole room next to the rear gardens where patrons could gaze up at the beautiful stained-glass ceiling and they provided settees and floor space so that you could contemplate the changes of colour and light without being rushed.

In this situation, I could simply be the same as everyone else, and this made me feel like I was normal, taking the pressure off having to get home quickly to lie down. It meant there was no opportunity for pain to interfere with pleasure, and it made recovery a *delight* and *not* a hardship at all. Tick. Tick. Tick.

There's always a list and for years now I have survived by being a diligent list writer. I have another dear client who shares this same affliction and we often laugh at ourselves, agreeing it's better to laugh than the alternative, and if paper were handy we would put that directly to the top!

The mix of drugs and pain often meant that my thoughts could get lost, so to counter this I had honed my concentration skills. At work, I would write down everything that I wanted to achieve with each client and then work around that plan loosely as they would often present unexpected things that required special treatment on the day.

Being flexible in this way allowed me to really hook into where the client was at, what they needed from me and what I was capable of giving.

Each client was so uniquely different. This was one of the things that I loved about my work. I was always looking and listening, watching and assessing. The back injury forced me to find an alternative way of operating with clients, because I couldn't bend or lift load. I was not able to be physically involved with personal training, so I needed to adapt.

Sometimes the smallest of movements brought stabbing back pain and other times being too long on my feet brought referred pain to other parts of my body. There were times when it was impossible to figure out why the pain was so intense and sometimes things did not add up to the cause and response theory. It's difficult to apply logic to pain.

Reviewing my Train the Trainer qualification helped me realise that clear direction was the answer. I had learnt to assess by observation and could notice the smallest of things without anyone knowing, so all I had to do now was to hone communication so that each person understood the directions given. By the end of a session there was often a smile of gratitude, 'I don't know what just happened, or how you did it … but I feel so much better thank you'.

Working this way was how I received the best results; which warmed my heart and made all the extra effort worthwhile.

It did however have an impact on my pain and Steve would say time and again, 'You have to take more breaks or do this differently, Poss. Look at you, you're completely done … for goodness sake start looking after yourself, instead of your clients!'

The voice of reason was not always welcome. I knew that Steve was coming from the right place and that his concern was very much linked to how the roll-on effect rolled into our life, because there was only a certain amount of energy and constant pain used up a great deal of it.

Work was structured so that there was always a lunch break and rest for me, however often dinner would not be on the table at night if it wasn't prepared beforehand, and of course there was the washing and cleaning. There were always plenty of lists being shuffled.

It was a constant juggle to manage pain in my everyday life, making this old back injury the subject of another book entirely. The balance was precarious and many times the overload came crashing down as the reality of pain will always win would once again ring in my ears and my body. Finding the balance was like rollerskating on a very slippery slope.

The Merits of Cake

Once I realised that everything I did came with a cost to me physically, I was able to negotiate with myself. My personality simply dissolved in the first few years after my back injury, because I was defined and restricted by the demands of pain. As time progressed and my ability to manage improved, I was able to open my life a little to receive some of the most precious of gifts. Gifts that I would never ever take for granted again.

'One two three blow' it was another birthday and as always, the highlight was the birthday cake. Since the twins, Malcolm and Jessica, had been born into our extended family our clever niece had managed to perfect the art of cake baking to the point where each year the stakes were getting higher and more elaborate.

It was a Barbie doll stuck in a huge pink icing petticoat and a blue tank engine of some fame and importance waiting to be devoured. After singing happy birthday and blowing out the candles at least six times it was time to enjoy!

The term blow probably isn't quite accurate because at this stage we were all in stitches as the huffing, puffing, spluttering and head bobbing began to get bigger, faster and more exaggerated until little Malcolm had set fire to his hair!

Cake is like magic. It somehow creates such excitement and expectation that it can be uncontrollable and if not careful near fatal for over-enthusiastic little boys.

The twins were adorable and we loved them to bits. It was the first time in our lives that we had experienced such contact with little people and already Uncle Steve had taken the role of silly Uncle Steve, throwing them around, hiding and making rude noises at any opportunity and generally running amok until he'd call time out.

'Uncle Steve's tired out and needs to lie down now.' It's hilarious to watch as both kids pause momentarily, look at each other and then hurl themselves at him 'stacks on the mill' where they leap and jump and roll all over him on the couch. All you can see is a tangled mess of arms, legs, bottoms and heads all mixed up with squeals of delight. It's one of the treasures of life.

A NEW YEAR 2020

The funny thing is that by then he genuinely has had it but loves it so much he starts up again and off they go until their parents finally call a time out to let Uncle Steve recover.

My role is less physical due to the back pain and sometimes I wish I could also spontaneously throw them into the air or lift them up and give a massive cuddle.

It takes all my strength to restrain from this and instead I gently squat down to kid level and give what I can there. Finding another way, as my Nanna would suggest. It is however such a joy to witness the unbridled happiness that romping with Uncle Steve brings.

Watching them play, instantly took me back to the rear woodheap, a little girl sitting quietly on a stump and contemplating why I wasn't allowed to go and play with the boys behind our yard.

My brothers weren't available to go with me and so I watched the activity through the cracks of the wooden palings, careful that no one knew I was there. If I was as quiet as a mouse, it would be *almost* as good as being involved, throwing the ball in the air and jumping as high as we could to catch it.

Covering my mouth I stifled a giggle, as the youngest boy completely missed the last and fell into the veggie patch. This wasn't so bad; at least I wouldn't embarrass myself in front of the older boys. Sighing, I quietly made my way to the water tank stand to see if puss was about.

Christmas 2020

Christmas Day was just myself and Steve. It was a relief to have made it. Coping with back pain in the lead up to Christmas was a struggle, but the biscuits were baked, the smoked trout was tucked safely in the fridge and there was simply no room to fit one more item. Each year our family got together either on the day or near it and everyone was responsible for bringing different items so that the load was shared. It worked well.

Whatever happened we always looked forward to staying with Steve's sister Catherine and husband Bill at their beach house an hour or so out of Melbourne. If we were lucky the weather would offer up some sunshine for swimming so that Steve and I, Sally, Michael and the twinnies could load up the cars and find our way to the nearby beach.

There'd be buckets, spades, blow-up boogie boards, towels, bags, sunscreen, water and cut-up fruit, tent, a few toys and not many hands left to juggle the kids and so they rode high above the rest of us on the shoulders of Sally and Michael.

'Can you see the sea yet? You must be able to see it being up so high ... ok ... what else can you see from up there?'

And so the day went. It was such fun, and we loved everything about it and even though I had to watch the activity, rather than be involved, it was such a pleasure to see Steve running around the beach throwing a frisbee. Poor Coco, their old poodle, didn't have a chance and would run backwards and forwards, time and again, in the hope of one day actually getting it in her mouth.

This was normal life for Sally and Michael and we marvelled at their stamina. The twins were full on but together they worked as a team, taking it in turns to look after each other and giving a break to get coffee when it was getting a bit much.

We loved the ease that we felt with this family, it was special. Each year Sally and I would bake a cake of some description, much to the delight of Michael who enjoyed anything sweet, and each year he would announce 'that is definitely the best cake so far' as he nodded for a second helping. And strangely each year they just kept getting better and more elaborate. Once again *Gourmet Traveller* had a lot to answer for, not only in upping the stakes but also the kilograms. Christmas was a celebration of everything and everyone we loved because family and all it involved meant the world to us.

Sharing food together and preparing meals was something that Steve's family really enjoyed and most conversations centred around what was being eaten or planned for the next meal.

Setting the table was a delight as Steve's sister, Catherine, always had the knack of turning the very simple into something extraordinary. I first met Catherine during my high school days and had been blown away by her sophistication. She wasn't around much because she was at university but instantly became the sister I never had, sharing jackets or tops she no longer needed and making me feel very much a part of Steve's family. She still dazzles today with the ability to make something out of nothing.

Celebrations of any kind were given the same unprecedented attention, whether it be using dried arrangements of leaves and gumnuts, wild flowers picked on her recent walk, or simply colour coding the table to a theme, it was always special. This Christmas it was gold, white and dark maroon with Christmas bobbles hanging from the light above the table and candles placed around the dining area to give a feeling of intimacy.

The twins in particular liked this detail and there were many attempts to blow them out, relight them and start the process over and over and over.

I loved sharing Christmas with Steve's family and because there were no longer any parents on either side, it was down to our small nucleus that was left to keep the tradition alive.

My brother-in-law Bill is the most amazing cook and being a retired doctor he had somehow transitioned all his expertise into delivering some of the finest meals I have ever tasted.

It was amusing to watch him spend all morning preparing the stuffing for the turkey as it was something entirely in its own category and would take far too long to list all of the ingredients he used, suffice to say there was always a bit of a tussle at the serving plate if seconds were on offer.

The turkey was another story. With the stuffing well and truly stuffed, he would proceed to close up as if still in surgery.

The neatness and precision meant that there would definitely be no scaring should the wound heal and none of the delights it held would ever see the light of day, until served that is. Such a wonderful piece of theatre to observe and even better to ingest.

Pre twins, Sally would somehow find the time to make a gingerbread house for Christmas. This was a real treat and quite a work of art. I can still remember the very first one, it was lined with roof tiles of liquorice allsorts, peppermint leaves on one outside wall, red raspberries on another.

Inside the house the door was open to reveal the floor tiles, which were Smarties, and a lovely little family unit, Sally, Michael and Coco the poodle, all standing up in the centre of the house.

There was foliage outside of course ... more lollies, more icing, and from memory even a postbox. A neat unit.

Each year Sally reinvented the gingerbread house and it was always such an exciting surprise to see what her imagination would produce. Then she had twins.

We all think of life now as pre and post twins. It's amazing how one event can alter the lay of the land, but life has been so much richer for it and seeing the wonder in their little faces as the fire was stoked 'Hot! Very hot' said with authority and hand stop movements always brings joy.

A routine check was now necessary under cushions and behind seats in case a Christmas bauble or two were hidden as a Christmas surprise and songs of cheer and goodwill were now somehow mixed together with 'the wheels on the bus go around and round'. We were all finding our inner child.

My role was to bring the smoked trout, toasted breads with rosemary and the dill mayonnaise that accompanied it, along with devilled eggs, Waldorf salad, some kind of meat, baguette, wine and leftovers from our fridge.

There would usually be a platter of cheese, olives, dried fruits and fresh fruit and breads that I would do either as an appetiser or desert if we were too full of ginge.

For the last couple of years I had taken to making smaller gingerbreads and ginger spice biscuits just to save Sally the pressure of another thing to do.

They were nothing like the houses of the past, but it kept the ginger theme alive and was easy to graze all day with coffee and ginge, as Steve liked to call them.

He had only to say 'ginge' as we were heading out the door to the beach and we'd grab a handful in a ziplock bag and enjoy them at the beach with some cut fruit.

Gingerbread

Ingredients:

½ cup firmly packed brown sugar

125 g butter at room temperature

1 egg separated

2½ cups plain flour

1 heaped teaspoon cinnamon powder

1 heaped teaspoon mixed spice

1 tablespoon ground ginger

1 teaspoon bicarbonate of soda

½ cup golden syrup

Plain flour to dust

Royal icing ingredients:

1 egg white

1¼ cups icing sugar

1 tablespoon water

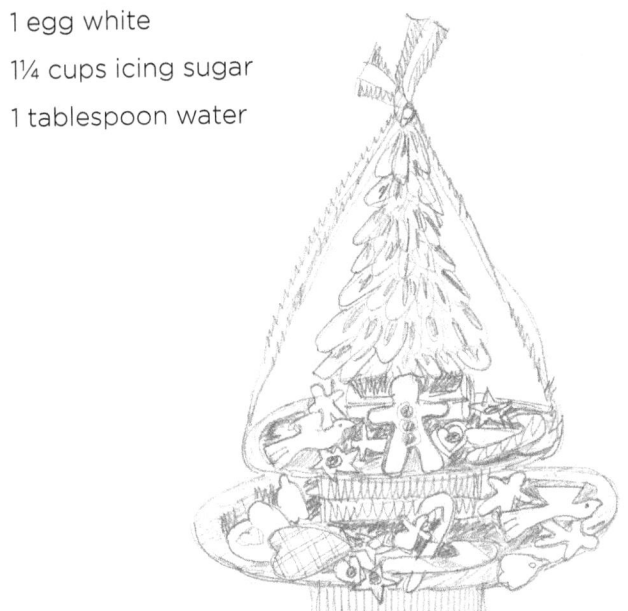

A CURRAWONG SOMERSAULT

Method:

Preheat oven to 180°C (160°C fan forced).

Prepare 2 baking trays with greaseproof paper and set aside.

Use an electric beater to beat the butter and sugar in a large bowl until pale and creamy. Add the golden syrup and egg yolk and beat until combined.

In another large bowl sift the dry ingredients.

Gradually sift them into the butter sugar mixture gently folding in the flour with a spoon.

When it has become a dough, turn onto a lightly floured surface and knead until smooth.

Press dough into a disc, wrap in plastic and rest in the fridge for 30 minutes.

Once rested, cut the dough in half and place between 2 sheets of baking paper.

Roll out until about half cm thick. Use any shapes you like to cut out biscuits. Bake in oven for 10 minutes or until brown. Remove and transfer to a cooling rack.

Method for icing (only prepare once biscuits are cooked and cool):

Using electric hand beaters, beat the egg white until frothy.

Add the sugar a little at a time and beat until soft peaks form.

Add water if too stiff; it depends on the size of the egg.

Spoon into a piping bag and use immediately as it will dry to hard and glossy.

You can decorate each individual shape with dots or stripes, anything you like, and then add Smarties, jubes or silver decorating balls on top to give a festive feel.

Devilled Eggs

Ingredients:
12 boiled eggs
1 heaped teaspoon curry powder
Pinch of salt
Sprinkle of pimenton (smoked paprika)
Mayonnaise

Method:
Place eggs in a saucepan of cold water and boil for 10 minutes.

Once boiled empty the hot water and refill with cold to allow the eggs to cool down gradually. (This way they shouldn't have any dark patches in the yoke.)

Once eggs are cool shell them and cut in half longways.

Carefully ease out the yokes and place in a medium size bowl using a fork break up the yokes until they resemble breadcrumbs.

Add a heaped teaspoon of mayonnaise to the yokes and mix. It needs to be creamy, so you may need to add another teaspoon. Add gradually, as the amount needed will depend on the size of the eggs.

Once mixed and happy with the consistency, add the curry powder and a pinch of salt. Once again be careful with the curry powder as you can't take it back but can always add more. When tasting to decide, wait until it settles in your palate as curry can be sneaky.

Place the egg whites in a large shallow plastic container with baking powder on the base to stop the eggs slipping around.

Carefully fill each egg white casing using a teaspoon to place and another to get the mixture off the spoon.

Once all the eggs are filled gently sprinkle with smoked paprika and store in fridge. They will store for about 4-5 days, and taste the best day 2 if there are any left.

Waldorf Salad

Ingredients:

½ bunch celery washed

1 white or brown onion (finely chopped)

3-4 Granny Smith apples (chopped)

80 g walnut halves

2 heaped tablespoons mayonnaise

½ bunch parsley washed (coarsely chopped)

Method:

Chop celery into fairly fine segments and place in a large airtight container.

Place finely chopped onion, parsley and walnuts in the container also.

Add mayonnaise.

Lastly, core one apple at a time and chop them to a similar size as the celery.

They will quickly go brown, so do one at a time and then immediately mix them into the mayonnaise mixture in the container so they stay fresh and crisp.

This salad will stay fresh in the fridge up to 5-6 days and will serve 4-6 people.

Other options are to add sultanas or boiled eggs cut into quarters.

Really enjoyable when placed in a lettuce cup to serve.

CHAPTER 15

Breaking News – Fire Crisis

We had been at the beach for four days and the forecast for the following day was catastrophic.

This meant that some decisions had to be made and quickly. There was really only one road to exit the beachside community and with the weather conditions predicted it would be deemed dangerous to stay, so we all left for Melbourne, holiday cut short.

Fire season was always a time of risk whenever heat and wind combined to threaten anything in its way should it ignite and everyone in the region had their fire plan in place and would grab their prepared bag should the warning be received.

A CURRAWONG SOMERSAULT

Gumtrees are in nearly all parts of Australia and even though they were loved by Australians and the koalas and birds who resided in them, they were an instant fire starter when hot weather dried their leaves and the undergrowth.

Once back in the safety of our city apartment we realised once again how vulnerable we really are to the elements. We watched and listened intently to make sure that those we knew in the affected areas were safe. The year had started. The warnings heeded. We hoped that everyone would be ok and that they would stay safe.

We had already been following the devastating fires in NSW, as they had been burning out of control since August 2019. Friends had evacuated numerous times and moved their animals to safer grounds. Not knowing just where the fires would hit and how long they'd have to evacuate was an exhausting and stressful process because fireballs were travelling kilometres ahead and causing spot fires all over the place.

Our friends Mary and Paul lived two hours from Sydney situated in the middle of national forest. They came to visit as they had a wedding to go to and it was such a relief to spend time together and see how they were actually coping. They showed us their fire app. It listed 27 out-of-control fires in the state and the fear was that they would all combine to form a wall of fire. This was real. This was very frightening.

We had met Mary and Paul many years before while living in Adelaide and we had shared history. It's rare to find friendships that remain constant over a long period and even though distance and other restrictions had reduced time physically spent together, there was a mutual bond that enabled us to pick up as if nothing has changed when we did. Mary was a down to earth, salt of the earth type girl who I instantly connected with.

We had both taken on the challenge of changing jobs late in the career cycle; I followed the fitness training direction and Mary joined the police force, working hard to earn her stripes.

For some unknown reason we had developed our own slightly warped sense of humour that sadly no one else seemed to understand. Steve and Paul would just shake their heads in wonder as we completely lost ourselves to laughter, crying, building the story as we went, getting more and more absurd as we workshopped an idea. It didn't have to make sense and that was the pure joy of our relationship. It was hilarious and such fun. I missed Mary.

It wasn't only based on humour. While living in Adelaide, the foursome, along with another amazing couple, had led and directed groups of underprivileged and troubled kids. Truth be known we were probably a similar age, but they didn't have the support or opportunities that we can all sometimes take for granted. So, as a team we took them camping, climbing, boating, travelling and provided anything that combined activity and time together to build relationships, trust and the opportunity to give support.

Over the years a coffee shop drop in centre was established and this provided a safe and non-judgemental place for these underprivileged kids to find an alternative way to be. Sometimes it worked, sometimes it didn't, but there were more positives than failures and it was worth the effort.

It was time for them to leave, and I stood at the front door reluctantly farewelling my dear friend. So many times over the last few years it has felt the same. The farewell.

It had done my soul good to connect with these friends, even for one night. Sometimes it's not the amount of time – just the time. The boys were on the street packing the luggage and Mary took both of my arms and looked directly into my eyes. 'You know what, my friend, you're still in there, I can see you … so hang in, I know you won't give up.' Tears hit. Mary knew my struggle, and without saying a word to her, she had understood. This touched my soul. It was the right thing, right time and something I would draw strength from in the days ahead.

Victorian Fires

Victoria was also in the middle of its own fire crisis. Smoke and ash were now a concern and the government and health

BREAKING NEWS - FIRE CRISIS

authorities were urging people to stay indoors if they didn't need to go outside advising masks were used for those with breathing issues or for expectant mothers.

The sky was blood red and dark, the streets were eerie. Very few people were out and about and if they were, then it was a quick process.

Hospitals were inundated with people unable to breathe and all ages were experiencing a whole range of symptoms from coughing, wheezing, sneezing and headaches to sore red eyes, and those with asthma were advised to use extreme caution. If this was what was experienced kilometres away from the actual fires, it was inconceivable what the conditions on the front line would be like.

My work continued to some degree, but many clients who were more vulnerable than most opted to stay indoors, in the hope that things would change soon. Weeks passed and we all watched the heartache that loss of life and livelihood brings.

The news covered all the detail and the vision was unbelievable. The acts of kindness, bravery and selfless fighting. Whole communities pulling together to share something, anything, even if they had nothing. Melbourne wept.

Giving money just didn't seem enough and Steve and I felt helpless and heartbroken. The year 2020 had begun in full force, with fire claiming anything in its path.

This was not what anyone had expected, and so far The Rat had not been true to its forecast of hope.

For weeks there seemed to be no birdlife, no other life at all. The air was thick, dense and smelt foul. With windows shut and no fresh air coming inside the apartment even the bedsheets and towels started to smell like smoke. Taking a shower somehow mixed the water and ash particles so nothing felt clean or refreshed.

It was everywhere and there was no escape. It was finding its way into the cupboards, into wardrobes and clothing and people were running their air-conditioning units non-stop just so they could feel like they weren't choking. We could hear our neighbours coughing and spluttering and knew at that point that they would be hearing exactly the same thing through their walls. Everyone was the same.

The white galahs arrived early in the morning. The squawking could be heard a long way off, but when they all landed in the street it was like nothing I had ever seen or heard.

They were a mass of white, hundreds of them fighting for position on the trees and branches.

Seemingly oblivious to what else was going on around them they jostled and squawked, upside down manoeuvres, one leg in the air, pushing, pecking and shoving, swooping and diving. The two large pine trees in front of the apartments looked like a Christmas tree stacked full of white ornaments with yellow crests, very heavy loud ornaments. It was deafening. I watched in amazement as they just kept coming until the whole street was aflutter with white.

There were feathers flying in the air, gliding aimlessly down to the ground like confetti. The whole feeding frenzy lasted about five minutes and then ... they were gone, screeching and squawking to goodness knows where. The mess was unbelievable.

Most of the leaves were over the cars on the street, and you couldn't see the pavement for the blanket that now covered it. Pine nuts still attached to their leaves were in pieces, discarded after a couple of pecks, and larger branches and twigs now hung at odd angles from the weight of their visitors.

The last time I had seen galahs en masse like this was at a family farm in rural Victoria, not far from where we lived. Pental Island was where my Aunty and Uncle farmed wheat, sorghum and sheep and as kids we loved visiting them. The land was dry and often resistant to being tamed, but we ran freely through the fields, played among the haystacks and chased the chickens to collect eggs, oblivious of Aunty and Uncle's struggle.

Years of drought and hardship brought a challenge to keep going. Wildlife suffered too, when food and water were hard to come by. Clouds of galahs squawked their way through the bare trees in the hope of finding something, anything, to sustain them. It was a sad and beautiful sight – once again nature had dealt a tough hand.

The Victorian fires had caused many animals to venture beyond their normal habitat. These poor birds were simply looking to stay alive. They were fortunate, they could wing it away. Others were not so fortunate.

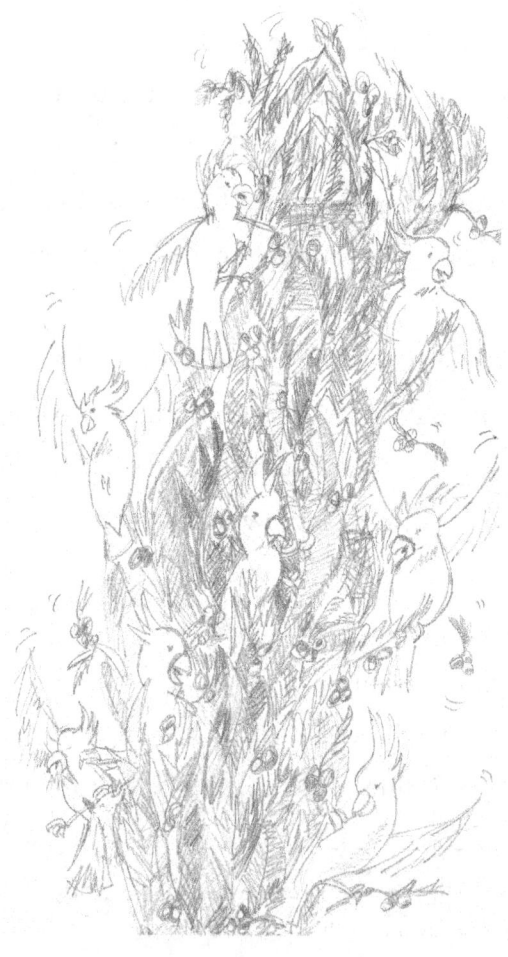

SUMMER 2020

CHAPTER 16

Summer 2020

The cool change arrived in Melbourne. At last! Not only could the windows and doors be opened, but it was now possible to go outside without the urgency to get back in and there were dogs everywhere, eager to sniff the wind.

The warnings remained in place, as the particles were still very much in the air causing symptoms to persist, but with the smoke lifting, the spirits of the city lifted with it.

The sullen sad blanket that had engulfed life was discarded and now you could see a smile here and there and eye contact could be made instead of rushing with eyes down to your destination. Lungs could be filled a little deeper, instead of the shallow breaths everyone had adjusted to. Faces were flushed with oxygen, trees gasped with relief and plants stood up proudly as they reached for the sunshine they had missed.

It's amazing how quickly humankind can adapt. When faced with a crisis or dilemma, bodies and minds seem to go into other territory.

> *'Survival mode is a short-term, fear based mode of thinking you enter when your flight-or-flight response is triggered.'*

Opening the blinds I breathed my first deep breath in a long while. My lungs welcomed the cool air and a coughing fit followed in recognition of muscles not used for some time. Who would have thought that breathing could bring such joy. I laughed at myself, realising that the alternative wasn't an option I really wanted to explore and, more importantly, I was looking forward to getting some sleep and pulled back the bed covers in anticipation.

Just the idea of lying in bed and feeling a soft cool breeze on my body made me feel so happy. This summer had been hot. It's difficult to remember the differences each year, but this one was uncommonly hot and a dryer than normal winter had contributed to the fire conditions that the state had experienced. Incredibly the smoke haze had not really gone but had begun a long journey around the earth's atmosphere to blanket other unsuspecting countries. Poor South America was wrapped in Australia's bushfire smoke some 11,000 kilometres away, with the highest levels of carbon monoxide in the world being measured over the clean South Pacific Ocean. Sorry America.

It's things like this that amazed me. The connectivity of the world and the environment is something I often wonder about. The cause and effect of things, and how sometimes the simplest of things can have dynamic and far-reaching effects. Oh yes, I knew about that. My injury happened suddenly, when I was at my physical peak in fitness and had never been stronger or more in control of my body and what it could achieve. How ironic. I now understood what it was to start from the bottom and slowly work towards recovery.

It took endurance.

It took stamina.

It took everything you had left.

Oh yes, the cause and effect of things could change the shape of life. It could be small. Very small. Almost nothing.

What looked quite harmless or insignificant could completely alter the turn of events, change the course of our lives or even turn the world upside down.

One moment in time. A word, a look, an event.

One simple action, or non-action. History has repeated the message time and again, when one person with power and position can wipe out populations because they dream of supremacy. Inaction can do the same when populations are faced with famine or natural disaster. Large or small the effects are far-reaching. At ground level we all have a part to play with cause and effect.

There seems to be a constant shifting and jostling with things, a readjusting of parameters.

It's like each person having their own unique force field around them. This idea intrigues me and I wonder what that force field may contain.

What would it look like? There would be past history and learned behaviours, perceptions, hopes, fears, prejudices, insecurities and assumptions all moving around looking for a place to settle or to be called into action at a moment's notice.

This force would be protective by nature. It would offer a supportive bank of reference to measure things against. It would shift and change, move and recalibrate, ready to offer a backup whenever there were interactions, conflicts or conversations.

A push pull, forward and back, like a child negotiating their first tentative steps. I knew I had something around me I couldn't explain because people often felt they could tell me things they had never voiced.

There has always been a willingness on my part to

SUMMER 2020

listen, but sometimes things happened that didn't make sense at the time, but on reflection became another gift or learning received.

'There's something there ... what is it? You have a calm energy about you ... is there such a thing?'

I was at a function seated between my friend's family, and had just heard for the first time that the young eight-year-old girl sitting next to me had been seeing a psychologist for over a year now. How could this be?

Such a well-mannered attractive child with very attentive educated parents. I watched the child and listened. I took her in and listened.

How could this be?

The child was quiet while her parents explained how anxiety had changed her from a carefree happy girl to a quiet and frightened one. I wrote something on my napkin and passed it to her when her parents were distracted. She took it carefully and then the pen.

It was a short conversation as there were only a certain number of napkins we could sneak from either side, but it revealed a loneliness that comes with high expectations.

> 'Softly, softly how does it grow? Gently, gently where butterflies land, opening, closing, finding a way, slowly reveal the depths of things you can't say.'

Everyone has a voice, it's just that sometimes it's not heard. And strangely, even though I'd never met her before, I realised I somehow knew that child.

Nowhere to Go
With my work studio located so close to home I was able to get there in no time and this was helpful if I had experienced a restless night and then overslept. It would be a mad dash but so far I'd never been late for a client because I always wanted to be there before their arrival to prepare and be present and focused.

Another plus was the quaint shopping strip just a block away which provided a wonderful mix of fashion, restaurants, gift and book shops and specialty grocers and delicatessens. Hawksburn Village had it all.

If there was a gap between sessions I would often walk up the street to get a few things to supplement the evening meal or just have a look around to see what was happening.

I really enjoyed shopping in smaller specialty shops rather than going to large cafeterias or centres, because like Prahran Market, it somehow felt there was a connection with the owner and I wanted to keep these small traders going so that they stayed in the area.

When you run your own business you understand the uncertainties involved and that income can change in a blink of the eye, whereas the costs associated are pretty constant and don't go away.

The day was sunny and I looked up at the sky to see white plumes stretching overhead. There was a flock of pigeons circling to my right making a wide loop around the rooftops and trees, and so I paused on the corner, watched them a few minutes and then obeyed the green walking man beeping to cross the intersection.

What a stunning day! Perhaps a BBQ could work for dinner and some salads? With a day like this the evening would be balmy and beautiful and with daylight saving now in place, sunset would be around 6:30 pm but the light would be perfect until 9 pm, ideal for the courtyard and a relaxed evening. Done.

As I walked toward the butcher I noticed there was someone seated in front of the fruit and veg store. It wasn't uncommon to see homeless people in our area and Steve and I knew many of them by sight, some were able to engage in some way but many were completely unable to respond due to the sad deterioration of both their physical and mental state.

The *World's Most Livable City* had it all.

There was so much to be proud of living in Melbourne. There were tea towels and shopping bags that highlighted the go see iconic landmarks. Trams rattled by advertising the latest Broadway musical or ballet, buskers entertained between market stalls near the Arts precinct, sports venues were packed with enthusiastic supporters and restaurants spilled onto the pavements. The Botanic Gardens featured a moonlight opera or cinema and music regularly echoed from nearby outdoor festivals.

We had it all – Melbourne shone in its glory.

But even as the national flags flew high and proud over public buildings, there was an underlying hint that *some* things that resided underneath were slightly out of place.

Coming out of the fruit and veg shop I stopped and observed the figure seen on arrival. She was slim, with short matted hair, her jeans were worn but reasonably clean and the oversized black puffer jacket almost hid her completely. She was huddled at the entry with both her knees held tight against her body.

A woollen beanie was next to her, holding a few coins. She must have known I was there because at that moment she looked up. Nothing could have prepared me for what I saw. The most amazing blue eyes I had ever seen gazed at me. Aquamarine. Flecks of glass hidden beneath them reflected something else.

Smiling, I said, 'Hi there.'

Once again I was surprised as I saw a hint of a smile on the grubby face and the eyes, the eyes said something, they said something I couldn't fathom.

SUMMER 2020

I knelt down next to her, careful not to obscure the entrance of the shop, and shuffled awkwardly to avoid being knocked by the customers going in and out.

'Well you've got a good position here, that was a good idea, how's it going so far?'

The young woman or girl looked down now, picked up a coffee cup and mumbled something about she had been given a coffee by someone. What happened next sparked the most remarkable conversation I had ever had in my life. Without hesitation I delved into my bag, pulled out my wallet and emptied the complete contents, paper and silver into the waiting beanie. 'That's all I have I'm afraid other than these bananas. I'd be most grateful if you would accept these as well?'

I placed the bananas on top of the now full cap and noticed the girl's mouth was opening and closing without any noise coming out. 'Are you ok? Do you need a glass of water?'

She shook her head and picked up the cap. 'Thank you, thank you, you have been so generous, thank you.' With tears in her eyes and fumbling she quickly put the money in her front pocket and then extended her legs. They were thin and the black shoes were scuffed and worn. 'You just gave me everything, how could you do that?'

I introduced myself and asked her name. Ciandra had just arrived from Sydney. It had been a long trip, a very hard trip to get here. Somehow she had heard that Melbourne was a good place to be ... the irony wasn't lost on me. She was tired but was here as part of some project ... this didn't make a lot of sense but I listened and asked an occasional question.

'Where do you usually hang out? Where do you sleep when the weather turns foul?'

She was constantly on the move. It was safer that way.

She often slept on people's verandas when lights went out. It was dry and she'd get a couple of hours sleep and then move on before anyone noticed.

'You know, I would have done exactly the same,' she said. I didn't know what she meant and so asked her to explain. 'I would have given everything too if it was me.'

I looked at Ciandra and realised that this girl was very special. 'Yes I can see that about you, Ciandra, I can see that in your eyes. You have very kind eyes.'

Ciandra smiled a half smile, partly to hide her missing and blackened teeth. She nodded her head. As she was new to the area, I mentioned where she could find the Prahran Mission and what they could perhaps assist with. She said, 'I probably won't go there but thank you.'

She spoke about a woman who had once offered her the choice of a room for the night or money. She didn't want to appear rude so she took the room.

She felt bad that she had trashed it. She had gone crazy being cooped up. She felt so bad for the woman who had only tried to help, but she was scared she was going crazy.

I understood. Weirdly, Ciandra touched a nerve. 'You know what, Ciandra, in some weird way we are all a little crazy, it's just perhaps some of us hide it in different ways. You're not losing it. You're tired, you're living rough, and quite frankly I can't imagine how hard that must be. I actually admire you. You are one brave woman, I couldn't do it.'

Something must have shifted, Ciandra was uncomfortable in her position and customers were pausing at the door, curiosity getting the better of them.

I excused myself and said it was a pleasure to meet her, that I must get back to work but that I would look out for her in my neighbourhood. 'Please take care of yourself, Ciandra – until we meet again.'

We shook hands and I wondered whether I would ever see her again. Walking back to the studio I felt different. I looked up at the same blue sky, observed the same white clouds, and realising that dinner would have to be more creative tonight, I looked to the sky to keep Ciandra safe.

An Idea Without a Plan is Just a Wish

It's a country wellness retreat. A place of sanctuary and healing. Somewhere to go when the pace of life has taken its toll, to regroup, rest, find yourself again.

Calm it down. Breathe.

A CURRAWONG SOMERSAULT

Good food. Chop the wood and collect the eggs, pick the produce and then cook together. Fill your lungs and allow time to sort out the stuff, to be yourself and relax.

I have always had a thought sitting in the recesses of my mind. Things often started that way – a dot – an illusion. A glimpse would appear randomly and I would look at it in wonder and then let it go, not really knowing what had just happened. Curious, very curious. It was as if there was another sub-story of my life running on a different plain which flickered snippets of ideas as a teaser, revealing only just enough to make me wonder what it all meant.

I have met and worked with so many different types of people over the years, each of them unique, and with their own individual needs.

I count myself privileged to be part of their lives and their world. It is easy for me to care for my clients because I hold them with respect and find so much wisdom to be learnt in what becomes trusted relationships.

Whether cancer or terminal illness had devastated the physical or self doubt and trauma have unsettled mental wellbeing, I am constantly in awe of how the simplest kindness given, so small you can barely see it, can touch a heart in search of reassurance or love.

To be cared for is a gift.

To give care is the ultimate gift.

SUMMER 2020

Over time I have started to see a picture, little snippets at a time. A place built around a large kitchen and a warm and inviting fire. Daylesford is part of this dream. I can imagine it as lush and green with places to go, nooks and crannies and places to be. Cosy accommodation that's private and beautiful; a place that offers peace, laughter, acceptance, mixing gentle exercise and stretch therapy with life and support.

This was the dream that was starting to unfold.

Could it actually be real?

In all my imaginings I can't quite figure out how it can happen. There have been many challenges over the years, most of which required me to work hard, very hard. I'm used to that and know that this dream of a rural retreat in Daylesford will need to be earned if it is to happen at all.

It seems out of reach, too good to be true, but it is persistent and isn't going away, so like most dreams, I have learnt to wait patiently, hold things close to my heart and trust that time in its wisdom will reveal all. Time will tell. Yes indeed … time will tell all.

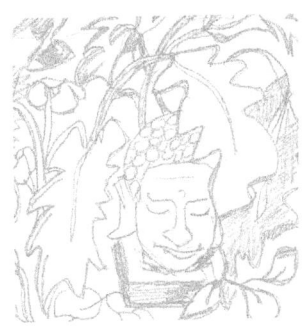

What Virus?

The 5th of January 2020 was the first time anyone had heard of the virus. There had been an outbreak of what appeared to be a cluster of pneumonia cases in Wuhan, Hubei Province.

The news was brief and to the point. China was a long way from us and no one gave too much thought to the news other than feeling sorry to hear that another virus had sprung up from the same region. SARS or severe acute respiratory syndrome had taken hold of the world 17 years ago and many people had forgotten the impact that this had had.

Time has a way of playing with our memories, we discard what is not immediately relevant and gloss over the rest, even though SARS spread to over 8,000 people worldwide and nearly 800 people died.

February was still fairly hot in Melbourne and there had been a few days where the smoke haze had created a pink haze over the skyline, just a hint to remind us all that it was still lurking around and we were not to speak too enthusiastically about breathing fresh air.

'You can't trust the weather, can you?' someone said in passing as she wrapped a linen scarf more securely around her nose and face. I smiled and acknowledged the thought while also adjusting my own scarf. I shuddered at the weather and saw how easily it had lulled me into thinking it was over and that everything had returned to normal-dom.

SUMMER 2020

That was sneaky, very sneaky indeed.

There would be no flights today, only more disruption for travellers and airlines. The skies were once again quiet and dark and cars drove with lights on during the day.

One step forward and two steps somewhere else.

A CURRAWONG SOMERSAULT

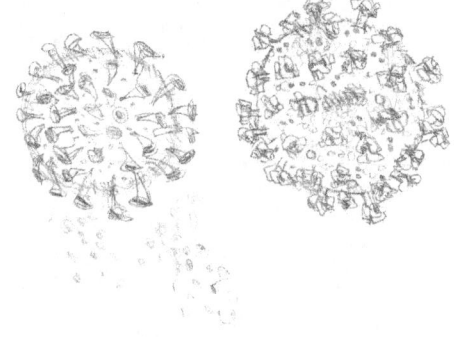

CHAPTER 17

COVID-19

'February 11th, 2020 the World Health Organization (WHO) announced the name for the new virus that was now becoming a worldwide threat. This coronavirus was called COVID-19.'

News channels were fighting for information to help clarify just what the world was dealing with. They showed pictures of round puffy circles blossoming into pink-red feelers.

They looked pretty. They were deadly.

The first case identified in Australia was in Victoria on the 25th of January 2020 when a man who had just returned from Wuhan, China, had tested positive.

Something had shifted, changed. All of a sudden China's distant news was very real and now living with us and the visitor it had brought on board was not a welcome one. Once again in the space of two months, Melbourne held its breath. This time the concern wasn't the air quality. This time it was contagion.

My clients were becoming more and more anxious. Cleaning had ramped up to the point that I was greeting them at the door, opening it for them and asking them to please wash their hands prior to commencing, then of course there was the hand sanitiser applied throughout and madly cleaning everything touched before the next client arrived.

Distance was respected and rubber gloves were used.

This was a different world.

There was so much talk. It was exhausting. The emotional drain along with the added cleaning was taking its toll on me physically. Pain was becoming more persistent and I was starting to feel uneasy.

Nearby Toorak Village had reported a cluster of the virus in a medical centre March 7th and there had been inconsiderate travellers who had not maintained the two-week quarantine period, therefore adding to the spread.

The world was beginning to unravel. It was a mad scramble by the health authorities to backtrack and locate anyone who had been in contact with this clinic and the travellers.

Numbers increased – countries were watching each other.

What on earth was happening?

Italy was in crisis and the footage was terrible. The sheer numbers of contracted cases and deaths stunned everyone. Hospitals battling under the pressure and lack of knowledge and respiratory equipment sent shockwaves through all health departments.

Were we safe? Steve and I didn't know. I could trust my own attention to detail with cleanliness but I wasn't confident in the awareness of many others I knew. Even those with the highest intelligence were not fully grasping the virility and threat that this new virus presented. One couple even had drinks in their garden with some friends who had been in contact with the Toorak Village COVID perpetrators.

They were in quarantine but deemed themselves safe to converse at a safe distance.

I was beginning to feel the weight of care and the duty I held for all my clients' wellbeing. Sleepless nights had led to a decision. I would have to shut my business to keep my clients safe, nothing else mattered than that. If I went bust, so be it.

And then it happened. Sunday 22nd March 2020 I listened to the Prime Minister of Australia, Scott Morrison, announce the plan that would hopefully save Australia the countless deaths that were being witnessed in many other countries. We were all going to take a pause in proceedings.

To shut down the spread of the virus we all needed to actually shut down our lives and stay home. He spoke with passion and clear determination and for the first time in his political history he was actually leading a nation. The outcome might be currently unknown but the consensus was that the alternative was death. It was now down to the basics. Life or death. The boundaries were reset because there was no negotiating with this virus.

It was now termed a pandemic.

And so it was that I sent word to all my clients. As of Monday 23rd March 2020 I would be closing my doors. I'd be in touch of course but wanted my clients to stay at home, do what was required by the health authorities and above all else, stay safe.

News and updates became the norm and COVID-19 infiltrated every crevice inside our apartment. Steve was now working from home and putting the finishing touches on the advertising campaign of a major property group. He was set up in the second bedroom/study upstairs and managed to maintain some semblance of routine.

The new normal presented a very different scenario for me.

I woke late and looked out the window. A massive crane had been erected directly behind our apartment and it looked like the crane operator may be able to see me from his perch so I opted to stay in bed. That was a good excuse if ever there was one, though Steve might not be so convinced.

Staying in bed was a luxury. I watched and listened to the hum of the crane as it moved up and over the rooftops and then it went down amid beeping and yelling. Someone had said something and then louder 'Watch it, mate!' and then there was an old fashioned telephone ring.

Fascinating really, the intricacies of the development site and its workings.

If I'd had my time again I often mused I would have enjoyed being an engineer or an architect. The idea of creating something from nothing and solving complicated problems appealed. I had to get up, I knew it, but what did I have to get up for? That was the question.

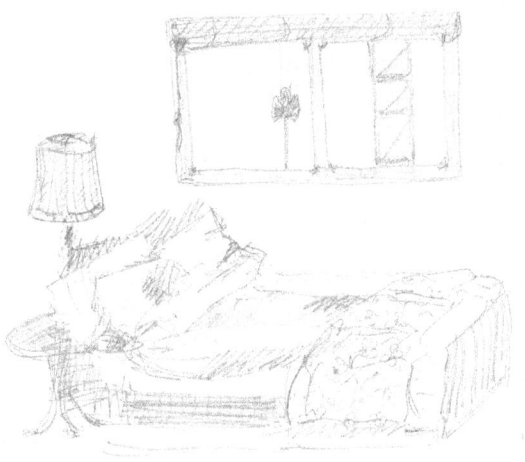

Clients were leaving messages, so many messages. Some were concerned about what the pandemic meant for them, others were just worried about the future and a couple were wondering how my business would survive. All valid in their own way but at this stage I had no idea what anything meant as I was as shell-shocked as they were.

The differences were very clear however; my livelihood and future were on the line. But their concerns and fears were real and they looked to me for reassurance and guidance.

Media announcements from the government were running thick and fast, with the lay of the land altering almost daily. We were all to stay home. We had to wash our hands often for 20 seconds. Use soapy water or sanitiser or both. Stay distant from everyone – 1.5 metres was the measurement. We were not to go out unless we absolutely had to. No interaction other than with the people you lived with. They were rules and they gave us something to do.

Rules gave a direction and a focus. Something to do to combat something we couldn't see.

For the first week I couldn't bring myself to speak personally with my clients, other than the ones that lived by themselves and were more vulnerable. I couldn't answer their questions.

It broke my heart and I didn't know what to do. Sometimes I'd find myself wandering around the apartment aimlessly, picking something up somewhere and putting something down somewhere else. *Ok, this is enough to drive a girl crazy, something has to be done, it's only day three for goodness sake!*

And there it began. The big clean had commenced and first on the list was the pantry from top to bottom.

I then was struck by a horrifying thought. I realised that if I contracted the virus and was isolated, there had better be a plan of action in place for Steve, otherwise chaos would break out. I could just imagine all of the pantry contents out while he was simply looking for the pepper.

And so the inventory commenced. Everything on every shelf was listed and recorded and placed in clear folders so he could see at a quick glance, what was where.

Pulling everything out to find something would now never be necessary. Tick.

Day five and suddenly there had been a strange rush on toilet paper. Great mystery surrounded just how and why this had occurred but all of a sudden a rigid panic took hold of Australia as a whole. Perhaps someone somewhere saw someone heap the toilet paper onto their trolley, casually shrugging 'you never know ... just in case'. Whether people needed it or not they purchased it. Loads of it. One man had filled a room with it and I was immediately taken back to what Ciandra had said and our discussion on different types of crazy ... now here was fact.

A CURRAWONG SOMERSAULT

Within the first week of lockdown, a flashback to the Depression or post-war restrictions had caused a stampede for flour, pasta, tinned produce of any kind, soap, tissues, cleaning products and all manner of weird and wonderful things that had nothing to do with anything.

I marvelled at the empty supermarket shelves where rows and rows, aisle after aisle were empty ... that was until you got to dog food or makeup.

Quite clearly no one was interested in looking good in lockdown and sadly man's best friend was not appearing at the top of the shopping list. Time would tell. Give it time, people can become predictable and I decided to watch those aisles with interest.

> *"We don't need to find a set up where someone wins and someone loses."*
> *– Jimmy Bonduc, 1992, 'Let Me Be the One'*

Supermarkets were reaping huge rewards at a time when it looked like we would never see food again. It was about survival, the base grade denominator. Fear was biting at the heels of many and the only way they could feel some kind of security was to stock up and look at it.

It did however occur to me that perhaps I had underestimated the eating capacity of those living around me. There were usually many pizza boxes and bottles stacked

COVID-19

almost in the recycle bins, but this was consumption at a whole other level, they spilled onto the ground around the bins, stacking up like pizza pyramids. Medals could be won if the Olympics ever considered pizza consumption a worthwhile sport.

March was silent. There were no racing cars accelerating around the Grand Prix track, no jet planes rattling windows and foundations making every dog in the neighbourhood go out of their brain. There was no buzz in the atmosphere, no diversions of traffic. Italy was in crisis with the virus and a member of the McLaren team tested positive. The talk was about closing borders and air travel.

The Melbourne Grand Prix was cancelled, only hours before the first practice was to begin. It was deemed too risky for spectators and competitors alike and so unhappy ticket holders stood around the perimeter gates with their passes flapping around their necks in the breeze, confused and fearful as they waited for the final decision. This unsettled Melbourne.

We were the sporting capital, this couldn't be happening.

We were all patiently waiting for the footy season to commence and the underlying fear that followed the closure of the Grand Prix sat silently in the room. No one dared say it out loud, to voice it made it real.

And then it was announced. 'The world and Japan would have to look seriously at cancelling the upcoming Olympics.'

It was clear that massive groups of people would not be able to meet.

Travel and borders were beginning to shut down, athletes would be put at serious risk and the overall health of the population had to be considered. What a shock.

For the first time in history the Olympic Games were postponed, due to the COVID-19 outbreak. After much debate it was agreed that they would be held from 23rd July 2021 in Tokyo. Hopefully.

The fall-out was huge as Japan had invested so much to get ready to host the event.

The media relayed stories of athletes from around the world who had relentlessly trained to be ready to perform on the world stage. They were lost and left floundering, not knowing what to do next. It was so upsetting to watch. Would they survive? What did it mean for their futures? If the Olympics were affected then many other events would be also.

Reality was setting in and it didn't look or feel good.

It was then that I heard my phone *ping*.

Please God ... not another question.

The last message had been from a client asking what brand of treadmill she should buy?

She was going to keep things going ... which was great, but after the next couple of questions only days apart, regarding the weight of the ball we used and whether she should get a bike also? ... I wondered exactly what the future would look like for my business. These were strange times indeed. People were not acting as per usual. I would need to be patient and realise that most were just trying to make sense of their new circumstances.

So as I gave information, brands and recommendations to many clients, reminded others of safe techniques to release a stiff back or troublesome hip and sent stretch routines to maintain status quo, I mused as to whether I would actually have a fitness training business when and if these restrictions eased. The government was now flagging that we should consider the possibility that things would 'never be the same again' and that we would all 'have to adapt to a new normal and live with the virus and it's restrictions'.

Once again time would eventually reveal all.
Once again it was a wait-and-see situation.
Once again no one really knew.
Ping ... Ping.

Humour at its Best

There is something truly remarkable and unique about the Aussie sense of humour.

Often sarcastic, our dry wit makes fun of *anything* and if you look closely it can be seen in our native animals. Have you *ever* seen such a strange and humorous assortment of creatures?

The kangaroo has enormous feet that look like elongated table supports bent at right angles. They stick way out in front of the animal ready to propel it quickly at a moment's notice. They jump. They can jump extremely high and travel very fast. A fully grown red kangaroo can clock up to 35 kilometres per hour, as their huge long muscular tail follows along behind like a rudder. Little arms and paws delicately hold food or scratch parts of their body as required and there's a built in pouch for females so they can transport and bring up the family very close to home.

The koala is a cute, furry bear-style animal which predominately lives in Australian gum trees. They are round in stature, squat in shape and have a large circular head with big fluffy ears and an even larger nose that seems to wrap around half their face. They appear docile and cute because they seem sleepy most of the time.

Most of Australia likes to think that they are drunk half the time but the truth of the matter is that the leaves they eat are so low in nutrients that they need more sleep than most animals, basically because it helps conserve energy.

The platypus is probably one of the strangest. They are a mammal that lays eggs. They live mostly in water and are expert swimmers because of this, using their flipper-style feet, long scoop bill and rudder tail to advantage when on the hunt for food. Venturing on land however is a very different story as they'll walk on their knuckles to protect the webbing on their feet. They can grow to 60 cm long, have dense brown silky fur and use electro-reception to find their prey and can render them stunned by using the venom stored in a spur in the male's rear hind foot. Charmed I'm sure.

Glancing at my phone showed there was a message from my friend Marian.

It was always great to hear from her and I had been wondering how the family were coping with the new restrictions. They lived about four hours away in a rural community and were actively taking over the family farm.

A somewhat challenging and daunting task for city dwellers, but so far the young family were doing a great job and were bringing up their two children Grace and Dean in the freedoms that farm and country life offered. Marian and Mark were a team.

They were younger than us, but were very much part of an extended family that had evolved over time. Marian and I often laughed about the simply awful life coaching course we had both attended years ago, but marvelled at how wonderful it was to allow us such a rare and privileged friendship.

Grace was my goddaughter and even though it was never formally mentioned, both Steve and I felt the same affection towards Dean, Grace's younger brother. They were special kids and equally so.

A CURRAWONG SOMERSAULT

The message flagged was a video. Trying to contain the giggles, Marian showed Mark and the kids decked out in their gym come disco gear doing a dance come movement instruction featuring the latest three government health requirements. Without any music, Mark in headband and American style accent led the rendition of 'wash-ya-hands let's wash-ya-hands' and 'san-it-ise and san-it-ise' and 'do-the-2-metres, do-the-2-metres' amid kids singing or yelling, as was Dean's contribution, showing the movements and getting faster and faster, louder and louder until Mark instructed the crew to 'break it down' and then they completed the whole thing again slower and in a whisper because they were completely out of breath.

It was hilarious and I played it over and over until all I could do was wipe tears from my eyes. Once recovered, I rushed up to Steve's Studio as it was now referred to and shared the love.

Somehow in a crisis Australian humour finds a way to cope. Across the board people were posting all manner of weird and wonderful takes on the situation and trying to offer a lighter version of the very serious situation we were all living in.

With so many people spending time at home, the streets were bare. We were seeing footage of ghost town streets, eerie and unattended: a shell in hibernation waiting for something to happen and spark activity and new life.

COVID-19

There was an ingenious jeweller advertising a $500 roll of toilet paper, which just happened to come with an exquisite diamond ring stuck in it. Fantastic.

Traditionally speaking, Aussies like to play around with language and have enjoyed creating slang or abbreviations for many words or phrases. Much of this is due to our playful nature but in times of crisis it's an effective way for us to lighten a very heavy atmosphere.

Not out of disrespect, more around the idea of helping us feel comfortable with difficult situations. So now the coronavirus is known as corona or the rona. A supermarket hoarder is referred to as a magpie. Hand sanitiser is now sanny. Isolation has become iso.

It's really no different to our love of footy, our need for a cuppa or that we drove through Macca's on the way home for some fries, instead of having a barbie for dinner.

'Jeez mate, did you see the bloke over there standing too close to the sheila who was doing a magpie with the sanny? Both of 'em should be in iso or sure as eggs they'll get the rona.'

I loved all of this playing around and remembered studying English literature during school. I wondered how *King Lear* would stack up if translated into slang?

Shakespeare was a language unto itself, so I added that to the list of wannabees I'd like to try one day. The list was getting seriously long in iso.

A CURRAWONG SOMERSAULT

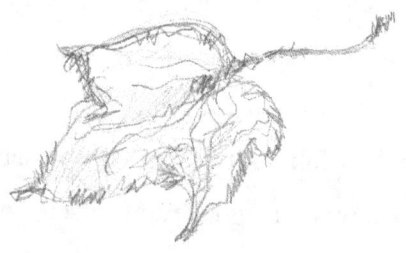

CHAPTER 18

Autumn 2020

It's funny how sometimes nature seems to have a switch. It's as if one day is sunny and blue and then the light seems to have shifted, slipped over to the right somehow, leaving long tendrils of sunlight across the courtyard as if testing physical agility to hunt for the warmth it contains. There's now a definite chill in the air and a crispness that makes noses appear red and cheeks a little flushed – that's if you're outside of course.

The large trees that line our street are showing hints of colour and looking out the front kitchen window across the road I can see the reflection of the massive crane working at the rear of our own apartment block. It seemed strange to be watching its moving arm go up and down and then hear the calls of instruction from the opposite direction behind me. A little to the left of that reflection, another window showed a more agreeable autumn display with leaves changing to yellow and blush reds.

Craning my own neck I tried to see the actual tree. Too hard. I missed being able to walk outside and feel the freshness of the air, to hear the crisp slightly damp leaves crunch underfoot, and welcome the comforting sights of the neighbourhood I loved so much.

We had fallen into the habit of having our lunch in the courtyard if there was any sunshine on offer. Not venturing outdoors into the world has made the courtyard the most prized position in our apartment, it gives a connection to space and even though it is enclosed and quite small it helps us to feel alive in some way.

'Let's pretend we are on the Riviera,' Steve says, as he tucks into the cheese platter in front of him. 'We could be anywhere ... we are so lucky to have this little outside space.' He then talks through all the plants he can see and the state they are in. 'These plants are in need of a haircut, those have grown so much ... but look healthy ... what was the name of that one again? Are all of these herbs?'

It doesn't matter that it was only yesterday that we had the same conversation.

AUTUMN 2020

All I can do is wait for it, nod and agree. It could be groundhog day, but it could also be a lot worse ... so once again the courtyard is analysed until we drift off into the possibilities of other things we could do with it and change the course of events.

The government announcements were coming thick and fast. 'These were unprecedented times which required unprecedented action in response.' It had taken a life-and-death virus to shake up political parties of both sides into working together to combat the situation and do everything possible to keep Australia and its citizens safe and alive. Watching this evolve gave us the sense that we were actually in safe hands and that the common good was now the priority rather than politics. Once again we were grateful to be living here.

For two weeks I tried to make sense of the latest government initiative, called JobSeeker. The idea was to financially assist those who had suddenly stopped working due to the shutdown and restrictions. Hot lines and websites were quickly uploaded to direct everyone to the right place and it was at this very same moment that everyone directly behind and in front of where we lived decided that they needed to get stuck into any home projects that needed to be done.

Our next door neighbours Andrea and Vincent had already commenced the reconstruction of their courtyard upgrade prior to lockdown but it was now evident that all the existing tiling was being drilled out of existence.

I had been on hold to Centrelink for 30 minutes and my ear was getting hot. Yes ... I knew they were experiencing enormous amounts of calls and yes I understood they were doing the best they could, and yes I would try and be patient but no ... I did not like the music selected as I was starting to hum along with something that after four days of the same ... was actually starting to raise my blood pressure!

For the hundredth time I disconnected just as the walls started shaking and my ears began ringing to the drilling of the world. Lucky that Andrea and Vincent were really lovely people.

These were testing times. The owner of the apartment beneath ours had commenced cleaning the outdoor tiles with a water pressure hose and someone on the other side seemed to be putting up a whole range of new artwork on their walls. We were completely surrounded by noise.

It was now week three of lockdown and I was still none the wiser as to how I was meant to get my customer reference number to apply for assistance if I couldn't actually get through to the department. All the while the news footage kept showing the Prime Minister saying, 'This will help everyone keep going when times are so tough.'

Oh yes? So far only stress, but thank you for asking!

And then a miracle, a voice was heard at the end of the line. I had tried a completely different government department in desperation and nearly cried to hear a girl called Sharon offer to guide me through the process of setting up my MyGov account.

During a lull in the ongoing renovations, I dutifully followed the steps, just so pleased to be receiving some guidance. It was at the end of this conversation that Sharon suggested perhaps I should actually look at applying for the small business assistance instead? She thought the new JobKeeper assistance hot off the press in the last government announcement would suit my situation better.

Not wanting to have to start all over again, I asked was there any chance she could direct me to the right department or, even better, a real person? Sharon went way above and beyond by transferring me directly to the appropriate department that would have a person attached to the number dialled. It was my lucky day!

The call rang and rang and then all of a sudden there was a woman's voice. I explained what had just transpired and asked out of courtesy to whom I was speaking? I was speaking with *Sharon* of course, another Sharon. This was too weird and after getting over the shock that the government only seemed to hire people of this name, I decided not to proceed with looking into a public service position.

Sharon number two was just as lovely and helpful as number one and I was at last on my way to receiving some kind of help, four weeks into lockdown. Thankfully both the freezer and the laundry housed enough food and toilet paper to survive so far.

New Life

There had been a few squawks heard but we were unsure. An unhappy cat? A new squeaky toy for the dog? Then we received a message and photo of the new arrival next door.

A darling baby girl had finally arrived for Andrea and Vincent amid the mild confusion of their other dogbaby Dudley, a very cute and lively sheepdog cross.

The whole family were fit, attractive and wiry so there was no doubt this little addition would complement the family portrait beautifully. Then there was a knock at the front door.

And there they were 1.5-ish metres away showing off the most adorable little thing you've ever seen ... and she was asleep. It was such a relief to get some good news!

I'd been worried that in being isolated during her pregnancy Andrea may have lost confidence in some way and been anxious because of the virus. One glance showed that any concerns were unfounded as the couple were tired yes, exhausted yes, shell-shocked yes, but they were very together in the moment. They were fine.

So I cooked. This made me very happy and was the only real way I felt I could be of any help. Restrictions were soon to be lifted for family groups, so until then, their family would probably not be on the scene for a while yet, so I cooked myself silly. The front door opened once again in tandem with the oven, letting all the smells waft around the walkway and the apartments below and then closed again with the changeover of pots and pans.

Buckwheat stockpot, scalloped potatoes and beans, Shanghai sticky pork with jasmine rice and apple strudel in filo with whipped cream.

Good healthy and not so healthy food that would nurture and reassure, support and sustain.

And then the cavalry arrived. The following week the family kicked in and the two eskies of frozen meals were paraded past the window. Vincent couldn't contain his relief. The back-up, along with easing of restrictions, had come just in time.

Apple Strudel in Filo

Ingredients:

2-4 Granny Smith apples peeled, cored and cut in 1 cm pieces

2-4 Red Delicious or Gala sweet apples, cored and cut

2 heaped teaspoons cinnamon

½ to 1 cup sultanas

30 g unsalted butter and 30 g melted butter for filo

100 g sugar

½ cup breadcrumbs

Sesame seeds

Filo pastry sheets and small glazing brush

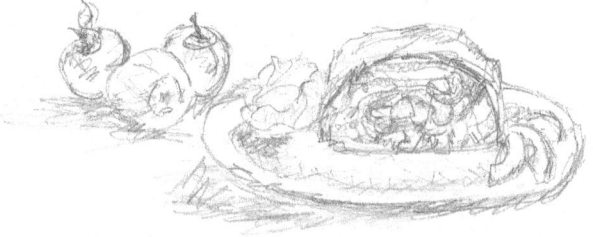

Method:

Bring filo pastry to room temperature at least 2 hours before cooking, but still sealed so it doesn't dry out. Put oven on 180°C (160°C fan forced).

Prepare 2 baking trays with greaseproof paper.

Peel, core and cut up apples placing them in a medium saucepan.

Add sultanas, cinnamon, 30 g butter and sugar and simmer gently until partially cooked. Set aside.

Melt 30 g butter in a small saucepan, ready to coat filo.

Check consistency of apple mix. If too much syrup gently add breadcrumbs. It should have some moisture but not be able to run out of the pastry.

Prepare a clean work surface with a little flour or instead greaseproof paper.

Take one filo sheet at a time and carefully brush with melted butter; work quickly to then add another sheet on top and brush this also. Cover the other sheets with a tea towel so the pastry doesn't dry out.

Place the apple mix in the centre of the filo pastry allowing enough space around all sides. Gently fold over centre and brush with butter, fold over the other side and brush, then repeat the same for both ends securing the ends. Brush butter over the parcel.

Sprinkle sesame seeds on top and transfer to a baking tray. The mix should make 4.

Bake for 30 minutes or until golden. Transfer to a cooling tray.

Serve:

Can serve hot or cold with cream.

Shanghai Braised Pork Belly and Rice

Ingredients:

340 g lean pork belly, skin on

2 tablespoons oil

1 tablespoon sugar (rock sugar is preferred, crushed)

3 tablespoons Shaoxing wine

1 tablespoon soy sauce

½ tablespoon dark soy sauce

2 cups water

Method:

Cut pork belly into ¾-inch thick pieces.

Bring a pot of water to the boil and blanch pork pieces for 2-3 minutes. This starts the cooking process and gets rid of any impurities. Take the pork out of pot, rinse and set aside.

Over low heat add oil and sugar to your wok.

Melt the sugar slightly and add the pork. Careful, it may spit.

Increase the heat to medium and slightly brown the pork.

Turn the heat back to low and add Shaoxing wine, both soys and water.

It's essential to have both soys as they give different flavours to the dish. Asian supermarkets stock all of these ingredients.

Cover and simmer 45 minutes to 1 hour until pork is tender.

Stir often, every 5-10 minutes, to prevent burning or sticking.

Once cooked, if there is still a lot of liquid, take some out of the dish and still leaving some, uncover the wok and turn the heat to high, stir continuously until the sauce has reduced to a glistening coating.

Serve:

Cook some jasmine rice to accompany the dish.

Steamed spinach or beans also work.

A month had passed in lockdown and there was a strange rhythm to it. I was getting used to sleeping in later if I'd had a restless night and the days seemed to merge into meals, planning for meals, cleaning, sweeping the courtyard, washing, Skyping, following up on clients, checking the latest health and virus updates and *not* looking at the bank balance.

April had commenced with rain. The forecast was rain and even though no one was going anywhere the idea of constant rain was making things all the more gloomy.

It wasn't supposed to be winter yet but Melbourne was receiving more than its normal autumn share, much to the delight of farmers who had struggled with drought for way too long. It was even filling up the water catchment areas, which was at least a reassuring thought.

Why do things often happen in threes? The first occurred a few days before when I decided I had better go to the studio to check the mail and any other goings on. I was all set, put the key in the ignition and was then greeted with a dreadful moaning noise rrrr..rrr..rrrrrmmppp!

It was cold, it was wet and that little car was not going anywhere. I rang RACV and amazingly assistance was not far away. Perfect, that was a bonus.

'Yes luv this is common with everyone in iso ... especially the older cars that don't do a lot of k's. Just keep it running for an hour or so and do that each week and it should be ok.'

AUTUMN 2020

Whew, another cost was definitely not needed at the moment. Things were getting tighter but the budget was holding it together ... so far.

And then strike two. The gas heating had been a bit problematic last year and seemed to like turning itself on randomly. It was always on the list, but the lists were long and somehow there was always something else that needed to be done more urgently. You guessed correctly.

After five days of wearing every warm piece of clothing we owned I reluctantly called a service man who confirmed its death and recommended a completely new system.

Steve was ready to donate his frozen organs to medical research and so in the interests of saving science the trouble of thawing him out, I contacted a service provider I knew and the installation was booked. How would we manage to pay for it? We would have to.

Somehow finances always seemed to *just* work out so I would trust fate and hope that the government assistance would soon kick in and help cover the expense.

It was such a relief knowing that we would soon be warm and cocooned inside our four walls. A sense of security was mixed with that and I realised once again just how fortunate we were to have comforts and a safe place to be.

Then I thought about the logistics. How were the men going to manage it all? The roof was two levels high and access was tricky. It was then that I also realised they would probably need to come inside the apartment to look at the temperature controller.

Nothing could have prepared me for the feeling of panic that took hold. It was brief and wild, like someone had just punched me fair square in the gut. That was weird.

I took some deep breaths and heard Steve talking loudly to someone upstairs. He must never know, this was stupid behaviour. My hands were shaking and so I sat down to finish the cup of tea and steady my nerves.

Face it girl, you like to control the safety of all and you just can't do that ... If they need to come inside they can wash their hands and stay at a distance, it'll be fine.

Of course it was fine, and the boys even took off their boots at the front door. The experience highlighted something very important for me though. Being in lockdown had also locked down my ability to be free and spontaneous and I saw my fear for the first time. I saw my fear for what it was. I was fearful for Steve and for all those whom I loved.

I was afraid of something unknown and invisible and realised that fear had nestled itself snuggly into my internal world. This needed to change. I decided that from now on I would respect the virus from the *very* warm comfort of our home and no longer fear it.

CHAPTER 19

Easter 2020

No twinnies this year. No Easter egg hunts or cooking marathons. No family get-togethers.

We were starting to really miss family and like everyone else on the news channels and specialty shows we were finding other ways to keep in touch. Connecting over dinner using Zoom and Facetime were such wonderful ways to still feel a part of life; a chance to really see how others were coping at the same time.

Steve had been a bit edgy and I was running out of ways to cheer him up so when our favourite pizza restaurant around the corner emailed a special takeaway Easter menu I rang and booked a delivery. It had been nearly a year since we had any kind of treat like this and I was so excited I tried not to give away the surprise by staying away from Steve. He was able to sniff out a surprise a mile off. He had the uncanny ability of reading me so well that it only took a couple of casual questions before he had all the info he needed. I would have to be careful. This would be a massive challenge. I stayed out of his way and put music on as a distraction, started reading a book and then began cooking. *That was a clever one,* I mused to myself. *He will think I'm just cooking dinner.*

So I set the table, making a lot more effort because it's Easter after all, and put a display of an orange rabbit on a cake stand surrounded with chocolate eggs of all sizes and varieties at the centre. The white and lime green theme was cheery and festive. This was fun and I felt happier than I had in a long time.

There was an enormous amount of chocolate as I'd planned to see family prior to the restrictions, so it was important to hide some of it in the hope that things would ease soon.

Does chocolate go off? I didn't know … it never stayed around long enough to find out.

The doorbell rang and the banquet arrived. Five courses of extreme yummy-ness.

Focaccia with olive oil dip and olives. Polenta chips with shaved parmesan and truffle oil.

Roast lamb and roast potatoes with rosemary and a cannoli stuffed with cinnamon cream.

EASTER 2020

As if that wasn't enough the lovely owner of the business had sent some hot cross buns and baby Easter eggs. It was almost too good to be true, and as we worked our way through the dinner we marvelled at the way something simple could completely lift your spirits.

It was worth so much more than just sharing a lovely meal together. For me, it was about reconnecting with my darling husband, dressing up and making an effort. Talking about something *other* than the virus and the upsetting way America was managing the health of its people. In that brief moment the virus had taken a back seat and life and love had cosied up in the front and we were happy.

Strike three. Of course there had to be one! This was unexpected however and no one was prepared to hear that the footy season was now in iso until further notice.

No one could believe it, there was always football, it was the life blood of Melbourne.

I was so grateful that the Easter celebration had happened prior to this announcement because we may not have recovered quite as well, if fate had dealt the other way around.

There was a numbness in the media world. They had nothing to say. What could they say?

There was no football. The world truly had gone mad.

And then the announcement arrived: 'With virus numbers normalising restrictions were to ease slightly, allowing up to five people who were family or close friends to visit at home.'

Whew!

This is what everyone had been waiting for: a reconnection with the world and those who meant the most. My dear friend Megan rang the day she heard; she wanted to come the next day. We had spoken nearly every day but to be in the same space was now going to be a reality and this was wonderful news.

Even though I was excited about seeing my friend I noticed a strange feeling lurking in the mix.

Apprehension? *Surely not* Anxiety? *Couldn't be* Fear?

No, I had dealt with that one already.

Firstly I had to check over the apartment, with my glasses on to make sure it wasn't slipping standard-wise. I only had a day's notice so it would have to be a very quick spruce. I also wanted it to be special for Megan as living by yourself in these restrictive conditions must be challenging, so I baked. Biscuits ... two varieties.

A cup of tea was nothing without a biscuit of some description and Danish ginger and Anzacs were two of Megan's favourites.

We could while away the afternoon and gorge ourselves silly. It was so easy spending time with Megan and now that our singing careers were behind us, we'd moved on to a sisterhood of sorts.

EASTER 2020

We knew each other very well and our history had evolved with us, as we both reinvented ourselves moving into completely different worlds. Megan in particular had truly gobsmacked me by taking on the IT world, a world so foreign to her that it was like learning a completely new language.

I can still remember Megan plonking the massive book of procedures on the table in front of her. She started work in a couple of days, and had to somehow get her head around it. She did of course, and has never looked back.

That was years ago and she had now excelled to the point where she was project manager for a number of large Australian and multinational companies. Never in her wildest dreams could she have ever have imagined that her life would do such a complete backflip. As we munched into our fourth biscuit we laughed about the way life throws up the most interesting of challenges and the fact that we had endured and survived *most* of them to date.

It was agreed however that this was definitely a bit of a tricky one. Its ability to be invisible and dangerous at the same time was certainly putting a lot of strain on our Wonder Woman skills. We smiled at each other bravely from the opposite couches, more than two metres away.

What a relief to be together. So much talk from psychologists and those in the know were estimating that many people may not actually recover from being isolated so long.

The thought that behaviours would change so much that emerging back into life again may take on a whole new way of interacting or connecting.

I understood exactly what was being said. Megan was the first person other than Steve that had stepped into our space to settle in and relax – our safe space. I had survived the installation of the heater ... surely I had moved on to higher ground?

In my mind's eye, I could still see the Skype interview with an Aussie man who lived in China and was in shutdown. This footage had come through early on into Australian lockdown but the message was clear. He looked down the lens and said a number of times. 'Just stay home, we've been in lockdown for 60 days ... it's ok ... it's better than catching the virus and dying ... just stay home ... you can't catch it if you stay home ... keep it in perspective. You have a home, stay there.'

We were six weeks in and that man's face and his message were imprinted front and centre in my consciousness. I looked at Megan. Her hands were shaking uncontrollably as she tried to get the sugar into the cup. This was not normal. I could see things were not 100% and that my friend had made an enormous effort in getting herself to my doorstep.

Some things you just can't pick up from a phone conversation and quite clearly there were other things at play. Megan rang her doctor and made an appointment. She was tough ... but even the tough can be occasionally vulnerable.

EASTER 2020

Danish Honey Cakes

Ingredients:

¾ cup honey

1¼ cups firmly packed brown sugar

3½ cups plain flour

1 teaspoon bicarbonate of soda

1½ teaspoons cinnamon

1½ teaspoons ginger

1½ teaspoons ground cloves

1½ teaspoons ground fennel

2 eggs lightly beaten

Icing ingredients:

3 cups icing sugar mixture, sifted

2 teaspoons softened butter

3 tablespoons boiling water

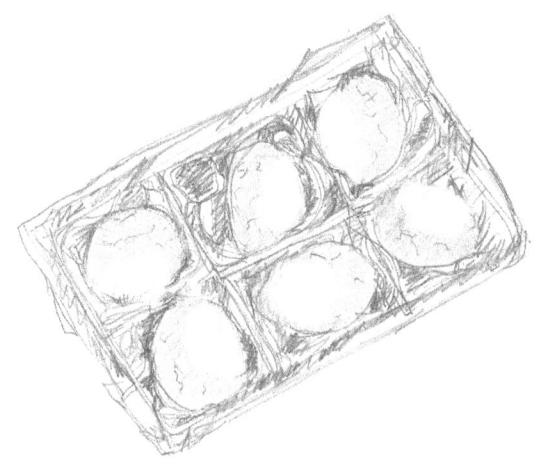

Method:

Preheat oven to 200°C (180°C fan forced).

Line 4 large baking trays with baking paper.

Place honey and brown sugar in a saucepan and stir over medium-low heat until sugar dissolves. Cool for 10 minutes.

Sift flour, bicarb soda, cinnamon, cloves, ginger and fennel into a large bowl. Make a well in the centre of the flour mixture, then pour in honey mixture and egg.

Mix with a wooden spoon until a soft dough forms.

Turn dough onto a lightly floured surface and knead until smooth.

Using lightly floured hands, roll dough into walnut sized balls.

Place onto prepared trays allowing room for spreading.

Bake for 12 minutes or until lightly golden. Cool on trays.

Makes approximately 50.

To make icing:

Mix icing sugar, butter and water in a bowl until smooth.

Top each honey cake with a teaspoon of icing and allow to set 30 minutes.

Anzac Biscuits

Ingredients:

1 cup rolled oats

1 cup plain flour

¾ cup desiccated coconut

¾ cup caster sugar

½ teaspoon bicarbonate of soda

2 tablespoons boiling water

125 g melted butter

2 tablespoons golden syrup

Method:

Preheat oven 180°C (160°C fan forced).

Combine oats, flour, coconut and sugar in a large bowl.

Melt butter and golden syrup and stir a bit (will look like caramel).

Dissolve bicarb soda in boiling water and add to golden syrup mixture carefully as it will froth up.

Pour into dry ingredients and mix to a sticky combination.

Put in fridge 15 minutes to set.

Line baking trays with baking paper and place 1 teaspoon of mixture allowing for expansion between biscuits.

Cook 10-15 minutes or until golden.

Cool biscuits on cooling trays and then store in airtight containers.

Makes approximately 50 biscuits.

A CURRAWONG SOMERSAULT

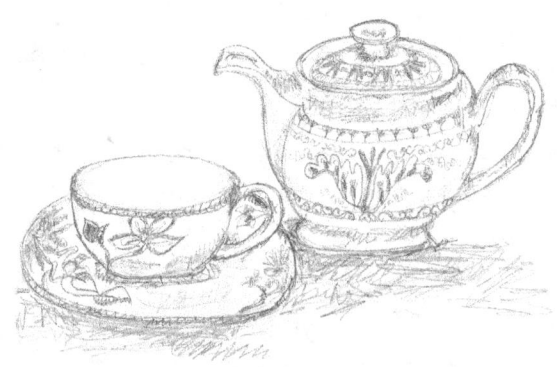

CHAPTER 20

Winter 2020

I once again listened to the rain pelting against the bedroom window. It was freezing.

It was winter after all and June was living up to its reputation as wind whipped against the trees outside, howling and thrashing through anything in its way.

The huge crane at the back of the apartment was groaning in resistance and still there were sounds of activity from workmen yelling out, though the wind distorted the sound, making some words muffled and others unrecognisable, carried away somewhere else with the wind.

They start at 7 am so often sleeping in is just a term for

resting while listening to the goings on. It's either the workers or the hungry baby's cries next door, but either way it's quite pleasant just not having to get up at that time.

I dozed. Steve was snoring. Mid-stretch I noticed the clock next to the bed was saying 9 am. Where did that go? I lay on my back gently doing the morning stretch routine, aware that Steve had already ventured out and was in the shower.

The rain had stopped and there was a noticeable lull in the outdoor proceedings, so it must be smoko as I couldn't hear any work activity. I loved this time of the morning, as I would gather all my concentration and focus on all the wildlife I could hear, and try and name the bird calls.

Gently rolling out of bed I opened the window slightly allowing a huge sweep of cold air into the room, shivered and made my way back under the covers. This was heaven.

Once settled, I could hear the little sparrows. How they survive such ferocious winds I would never know. There was a magpie warbling in the distance and of course a couple of crows nearby; that was always the case. Nothing else. I waited patiently.

I had a sip of water and nestled back under the covers.

It was then I heard it.

I listened, holding my breath. It was a currawong. I loved these birds and knew their call thanks to Bill's handy instruction book and the flocks of them that lived around his property.

This was different, however. I listened and listened. Smiled.

'Dwoh dwoh dwoh.'

Laughed out loud. Well there you go, it was a currawong there was no doubt about that, but the call was different to anything I had previously heard. Instead of droning on one note this particular bird was singing a major third. I sang the notes and yes it was definitely major not minor and the notes were 'E, E, C'. Gosh my jazz piano improvisation teacher in Adelaide would have been suitably impressed that I'd figured that one out.

I couldn't help smiling because he was the only person I had ever met who could tell what key a lawnmower was operating in and be distracted if it wasn't consistent.

After a few rounds of the currawong song echoing further into the distance there was another surprise.

A reply. Somewhat closer and obviously in need of a rendezvous, the unmistakable 'dweh dweh … dweh' rang out, slightly less confident than its mate. I couldn't believe it, and sat up on my elbows shaking my head and yes … there it was again … the complete reverse to the first call … 'C, C, E'.

I laughed in disbelief.

Sometimes life can give the best gifts when you least expect them, and here was one of the best. I felt I had just received something I could never explain.

What magnificent birds. They were freaks, renegades. They were tired of conforming to the usual currawong routine and had broken the mould. Perhaps they had escaped the conventions of wealthy beach living and ventured their new groove in the inner-city precinct. Perhaps none of the other flock understood what they were saying and so they had to move on and find a new way? Whatever the reasons I was very pleased indeed.

This was another welcome guest to the neighbourhood bird exchange and I would be listening out for them now that I knew their call.

Zoom and the Big Bake

If there was ever a buzz word of the times it was Zoom. Whether it was for scheduling work meetings, organising bridge nights, just drinks with friends or staying in the loop with family, it had taken over the world as we all knew it. It allowed a casual link up with others and reconnected the links that were missed so much. Friday 2 pm was the big Bake up Zoom meeting. Steve kindly set up the logistics of the laptop on the wooden pedestal and co-directed the kitchen angles to show my best angle on the receiving end. 'Steve, can you do something about the dreadful light around the eyes? And what about the neck? The stripe down the middle of the hair line looks a treat can you lift the camera higher to hide that?'

Poor Steve. There's only so much you can do, so I opted

to try some makeup, if I could find it, and donned the black apron over the black T-shirt and black jeans. Very black and very Melbourne. All the ingredients were measured and ready, with baking trays greased and lined, oven turned on.

Front door ready to be opened at a moment's notice.

Recipe. Done.

And so it began. I viewed the group gathered in the kitchen so far away. Grace, Dean and Marian were all decked out with pinafores and aprons of varying sizes. Dean's in particular made me giggle as it was way too big for him but he pranced around to show it off. Quite clearly this would make the world of difference to his baking skills.

And then theatre commenced as he took centre stage and started to read through the directions, giving everyone instructions as to what to do and when. This little five year old had spunk, he was adorable. Once he had broken the eggs and made a mess of the flour, he had exhausted all of his concentration and then proceeded to build a train track around the rest of the bowls and ingredients, more interested now to show off his vast array of trains.

I had never seen so many trains and they were now zooming around a track that circled the whole cooking surface. This activity made me feel that perhaps my kitchen was lacking in some way and so it was decided that perhaps Grace should steal a little limelight and read her latest story. So while the muffins cooked the story unfolded ... an old married couple who had a dog who was loved so much that he had numerous pieces of clothing made for him by his owners ... mmmmm ... oh yes?

As I listened to the story, I wondered whether COVID had perhaps awakened the need for another pet? The family already had a cute, smoky coloured cat. As I winked at Marian I could see this was landing on deaf ears, but it was very entertaining, nonetheless.

And then we were finished, amid laughing and chatting, checking and listening. The muffins smelt amazing and as the blueberry and coconut wafted out into the walkway area, I knew I'd deliver some to the little family next door before they cooled. After a quick wrap up and clean-up of the train station and work station we all waved farewell until the next exciting bakeathon. Such fun with all the people I loved the most.

Perhaps zucchini fritters would work well for the next exciting episode? I would need to hunt through my notes and check that they were kid friendly.

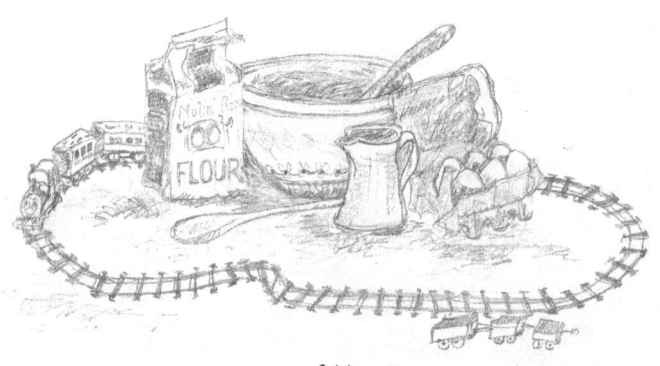

Blueberry and Coconut Muffins

Ingredients:

2 cups self-raising flour

½ cup coconut

¾ cup caster sugar

60 g melted butter

¾ cup milk

2 eggs (room temperature)

100 g fresh blueberries or raspberries (can be frozen)

Method:

Preheat oven to 190ºC (170ºC fan forced).

Line muffin tins with paper cases.

Sift flour into a large mixing bowl.

Add coconut and sugar and mix together, making a well in the centre.

Melt the butter and combine in a jug with the milk and eggs.

Add milk, egg, butter mixture to the flour mixture and stir until combined.

Gently fold through the blueberries or raspberries.

Spoon mixture evenly into muffin cases, filling about halfway.

Bake for about 20–25 minutes or until a skewer comes out clean.

Cool on a wire rack.

Makes 12 muffins. Can be frozen.

Zucchini and Mustard Fritters

Ingredients:

2 eggs

¼ cup self-raising flour

1 tablespoon seeded mustard

3 zucchini (courgette), 2 thinly sliced and 1 coarsely grated

2 tablespoons olive oil

Lemon wedges to serve

Salt and pepper

Method:

Place the eggs, flour, salt, pepper and seeded mustard in a bowl and whisk to combine.

Add the sliced and grated zucchini and stir to combine.

Heat the oil in a large non-stick pan over medium heat.

Cook ¼ cupfuls of the mixture in batches for 2–3 minutes each side or until golden.

Drain on absorbent paper.

Makes 6 and can be frozen.

It's worth doubling the mixture and having them cold another day.

Serve:

Try making a tomato, basil and red onion mix by chopping all ingredients into cubes.

Place a couple of slices of avocado and put the tomato mix on top.

Alternatively you can use avocado and smoked salmon with some fresh dill or chives and lemon wedges.

When in Doubt – Bake

The virus thrives in winter and it likes to attach itself to things. It's sticky and hangs around for between three and five days depending on the type of surface. It falls in droplets to the ground.

Its droplets can be dispersed by simply breathing or coughing or sneezing. Touching something that has been infected is a known trademark of its transmission. It's a tricky, sticky customer that sneaks around and even the best eyesight in the world cannot see it in natural light.

It's elusive. Imaginative. It doesn't like to show itself, until it's ready to do so.

So cunning is the virus that it can infect humans unknowingly. There can be symptoms, or no symptoms. Clever, very clever indeed.

The 1st of June 2020 was noted as being the coldest day on record since 1943. Melbourne was freezing. The wintry blasts threw all the seed pods from the silver birches behind the courtyard into every crack and crevice, confirming that these trees have to be the most prolific reproducers known to man.

I'd already swept up three bags of them and it wasn't yet lunchtime. If even half of the seeds took hold and sprouted, there would be no more concerns about greenhouse gasses, as we would be living in a dense forest.

The wind was howling and the graziers would definitely need to heed the warnings and tie down their sheep in this weather.

The thought brought a smile, as I imagined them tied to trees and shrubs, fences and postboxes. Oh I really should get out more. Oh that's right, I can't. What a shame the wind and rain couldn't simply blow the annoying virus away.

It did amaze me however, that such a robust virus could be brought to its knees quite simply if it couldn't circulate.

The stay-at-home routine did appear to be stopping it in its tracks, and the fact that lots of soapy water and sanitiser were its number one enemy somehow seemed like a weird twist.

Did this virus have a sense of humour?

If so, it wasn't very amusing.

It was a bit like Superman being rendered powerless by the use of a feather, instead of kryptonite.

> *"A sense of humour is the best indicator that you will recover, it is often the best indicator that people will love you. Sustain that and you have hope."*
> *– Andrew Solomon, 2000, The Noonday Demon –*
> *An Atlas of Depression*

The slow cooker was working overtime. Megan had kindly given this as a Christmas gift, and so far it was going well because the shoulder of lamb was slowly doing its thing with the potatoes, carrots, celery and thyme and Steve had been downstairs a couple of times already, in the hope that there may be something ready to sample.

That was the joy of an upstairs apartment, all the smells wafted straight up to Steve's nose.

Another four hours to go. This was going to be a huge test and I had a feeling I'd better put together a small platter of nibbles to keep us both going, or there would be trouble.

Apple, cheese, dried nectarines and walnuts saved us, as we tried to ignore the delicious smells that were now causing the neighbourhood dogs to sniff and scratch the door as they went past on their daily walk.

Dinner at last. I almost felt I should apologise to our neighbours for the aromas, as 10 hours was a long haul for anyone to endure. At least there wasn't too much chilli with this bake because sometimes the neighbour's garlic/chilli combination brought tears to my eyes. They must have stomachs of steel, or perhaps they have built up their tolerance over a period of time and now need the whole packet to register a shot of flavour.

It's a bit like when you have a shower on a freezing cold morning. It starts off feeling just nice and then you think ... *Oh maybe just a little warmer ... and a little more ... oh it's so lovely and warm ... just a touch more heat,* until by the time you step out to towel yourself off, you resemble a cooked beetroot.

We sat at the kitchen table enjoying the meal as if it was the one we had been waiting for all our lives. The meat fell off the bone as the recipe said it would, and there was true happiness in our little world. Steve marvelled at the way I had managed the meal and commented that I no longer needed his assistance to get things in or out of the oven.

It pays having another pair of observant eyes around. It also pays to acknowledge positive change when it happens and I was grateful that he had noticed.

In the next breath he declared how fortunate that the back injury happened when I was at my fittest.

'Gosh Poss, imagine if it had occurred when you were singing? There's no way you could have continued that career with pain.'

The mind boggles, and mine was now truly boggled.

He was right of course, singing involves every aspect of a person: mind, body, emotion and spirit. How fortunate I was that my gift of singing had not been affected by or associated with pain.

Scanning back over the years took me to where my singing career had begun and I shuddered as I realised just how lucky I was. We listened to our own thoughts and were oblivious to the newsreader in the background announcing that Australia was now officially in recession.

CHAPTER 21

A Songbird

Being in the church choir as a young girl required stamina. Somehow I was recruited without being involved in the conversation and simply fell into the routine of rehearsals, soon finding myself grouped with two other girls, and being known as a soprano. The choir fluctuated in numbers and could range between 12 children to a total of 20, which included adults. At eight years of age I was one of the youngest and I was positioned next to Debbie, who was a couple of years older than me.

Debbie Watson was very sophisticated.

She had naturally wavy brown hair, which she was allowed to

wear without hair bands, and she always dressed immaculately. She was confident, friendly, wore a bra and always sang very loudly.

She was an alto and it took all my concentration to stay on my own notes when standing next to her. Singing was complicated at the best of times, as there were notes of different lengths that sometimes went with a word and other times they were just held for the sake of it.

It took a lot of breath to get all the notes and words out at the same time, and I had to squeeze the air out of my lungs, sometimes feeling like I might turn inside out with the effort. If the choir was at capacity, and I felt I may be about to faint with the lack of breath, I would sneak a little one between the shorter connecting words, in the hope that no one would notice. A sneaky little breath without going red in the face.

"Jesu Joy of Man's Desiring."
–*J. S. Bach, 1716, Cantata 147*

This hymn was one of the most beautiful things I had ever heard. The introduction was like a gentle stream of water, making its way over different size rocks and pebbles. Rising and falling, it swayed the grasses at the edge of the bank, so that they moved in unison, smoothly and freely, just happy to be involved, even though they didn't go anywhere themselves.

It was the delicate melody that brought tears to my eyes. I

couldn't explain it, but as I listened, it touched somewhere deep inside, and made me feel that this was written especially for me. I'd sniff and blink tears away, reach for a handkerchief and avoid eye contact with the choir mistress until I'd regained my composure.

From my youth, music seemed to speak directly to my soul. I didn't know or understand what was happening to me or why, but I allowed it to happen. It seemed the natural thing to do, as it was something I felt I had no control over.

Sometimes there would be one particular line which was troublesome. Mrs Symonds, the choir mistress, had a very good ear and could pick a fudged note anywhere, even in the middle of a four-part harmony sequence with accompaniment.

She was an amazing woman, tall, wiry, with deep brown eyes that shone when she smiled.

I loved the way she looked just before the choir commenced singing. She would gather her music, set up at the front of the choir stalls, and look at absolutely every single person individually.

When eye contact was made, and she was satisfied that she had everyone's attention, she would mouth some words which related to the opening phrase, lift both her arms so that her fingers were held in front of her, place her thumbs and fingers together, take a deep breath, lift one eyebrow … and then it began.

We followed her hands, we followed her breath. We lifted volume when she did, we raced through fields when she felt we should go faster, and then we would hush to a whisper, when the words were too special to speak. The note which resembled an oblong circle, was held … and held and held until all faces glowed bright red. We travelled high, we travelled low. We were the music. We were the melody.

And then the accompaniment resounded with all the harmony building, soaring, until at last we were brought back to where we started. All eyes looking, wider now and waiting. Breathless and happy, both her hands were now back together, we watched and followed. An eyebrow signalled the close was coming, a sweep of hands in a small circle and then, and then … and then we were done.

What a relief to sit down and rest. Sometimes it was silent for a while after the choir finished as if the stained-glass windows were filtering the thoughts of the congregation. A couple of times there was applause. I was always lost for words and humbled. I felt blessed in some way.

Near Enough is not Good Enough

I had no recollection of whether this was ever said out loud. I wasn't even sure whether I understood the full implications, but what I *did* know was that I needed to give my best to anything I tried to do.

There was an invisible measure somewhere and it was set from the beginning of time, as I knew it. From an early age I realised that there was expectation.

By the age of sixteen, I'd completed Preliminary – Grade 8 for piano and theory of music with the Australian Music Examinations Board (AMEB) and Grades 1 – 6, including Elementary Level exams with the Australian Ballet Royal Academy of Dance, Checcetti method.

I worked hard. Practising piano before and after school meant fitting in school homework around the busy schedule. Some mornings were so cold I'd soak my frozen fingers in a bowl of hot water next to the piano, just so they could function.

In summer, the old fan rattled beside me, unable to stop the dripping sweat making fingers slip and slide over the keys. Ballet required three lessons per week and two for Piano and Theory tuition, often travelling two hours to Bendigo for the higher grades in piano and ballet.

There was always encouragement and support, a smile, a hug. In later life, I was sent all the newspaper clippings from my mother, all the photos and write ups of my performances, including copies of the TV shows that had been recorded.

The strange thing was that I didn't need to keep all of these things, I never looked at them, and certainly didn't talk about what I was doing. I just did my best at the time, and treasured the moment for what it was.

A performance was simply that. It required an enormous amount of preparation and work to get to the stage of presentation. The voice was an instrument after all, and needed to be cared for respectfully, so that it could maintain rigorous use. To develop a nodule in the throat was a singer's worst nightmare, something I wanted to avoid.

Choir rehearsals were held twice a week. I rode my little blue pushbike to the church at 8 am every Friday morning, before school. Sometimes the wind was so strong I would have to stand against the force, raincoat flapping around my legs, sticking to them in the rain. Other times, the air was so dense with heat I could barely move my legs to keep the bike from falling over.

Rain or shine, I attended, my face either completely drained of colour or flushed red. There were no excuses and I didn't want to let anyone down, especially Mrs Symonds, the choir mistress. The other rehearsal was after school on Tuesdays and this rehearsal was my favourite, as it was held at Mrs Symonds' home. She lived a couple of blocks from where my family lived, so it was easy to call in on the way home from school.

A SONG BIRD

Three girls would often be there. Debbie and Carol were both altos and I was the soprano. On arrival, Mrs Symonds would bundle everyone into the kitchen, where we would enjoy a steaming hot cup of milo and some leftover white bread crusts, smothered in butter and vegemite. This was such a treat. Mrs Symonds was a firm believer that no one could sing properly without sustenance.

We were very grateful. She made us feel very special.

Mrs Symonds would sit at the piano and play the introduction, followed by each separate harmony. Once we had an idea of what we were doing, she would ask us to sing our parts individually and then gradually add them together. Sometimes things came together quickly, and other times we had to go over and over sections, until we were completely exhausted.

'Let's take a moment, I've noticed something. It's not just about how much air you take into your lungs ... I can hear you're taking such big breaths to try and make it to the end of the phrase ... it's also about how you control the breath coming out.'

This was one of those moments in life where I was momentarily stunned. It was similar to the two flag umpire scenario that I'd become aware of recently, a shining moment, when all of a sudden I was aware that singing involved not just the breath coming *in*, but also how the breath came *out*.

The breath was the key.

The key was the breath.

And I was the one who controlled the breath.

I laughed and looked at Mrs Symonds, who was smiling.

I understood completely. This information had changed my world. Instead of fighting with my breath, I now started to listen to how it escaped me.

It was fun. It was weird.

Breath was sometimes like an uncontrollable force, untamed and with a mind of its own.

Other times I could guide it effortlessly over notes, and hold it longer than I could ever have imagined. Over time, with hours of practice, I began to understand how sensitive breath was.

It needed to be coaxed and encouraged.

It needed patience.

I learned to be gentle with it.

I learned to be demanding of it.

I got to know breath, and we became friends.

Finding my Voice

'It's only one song and would mean the world to us ... please say yes ... it's our favourite song ... oh please ... we've booked a band and they've said it would be fine.'

I wasn't exactly sure how Sally, my niece, had come up with

the idea, but after years of retirement and a genuine hint of uncertainty, I agreed to sing at her wedding.

'You're Just Too Good To Be True' by Frankie Valli was to be sung as the bridal waltz, after the main course and just before dessert. What could I say? I was already included in the program.

It's always a privilege to sing. There's a connection that happens deep within a performer, when exploring through melody and intonation what the composer is trying to express.

Like anything that requires self-expression, singing can touch souls. In the same way, music can filter through all our barriers and go straight to our heart.

Both expressions have the power to not only touch us but also speak to us in words that can't be described.

Rehearsals commenced, fortunately there was plenty of time, so I started a gentle warm-up.

It was my day off and Steve was at work, so I had time and space to find out exactly where my voice might be.

Most of the neighbours worked, so I felt confident that I wouldn't be causing them any discomfort. The scales were rusty.

Notes were missing. There was a huskiness I didn't recognise, and I was beginning to wonder whether this voice actually belonged to me.

I reminded myself that there was time.

Be patient, there was time.

Week after week I practised. Not the song ... but the voice. It was stubborn. It had been enjoying hibernation for many years and had settled comfortably into speaking mode.

Singing mode was not keen to cooperate and I soon realised that the best thing I could do was to relax, keep practising, and hope it would all come together on time.

Near enough is not good enough

After two months of vocal practice, I started working on the song. I had a month to hone it, and was starting to feel that perhaps it wouldn't be a complete disaster.

I was amazed that such a young couple had chosen a song like this. It said so much about them. Sally and Michael had met as teenagers and had developed a strong friendship, which reminded Steve and me of our own partnership. There were parallels, but the main thing that was evident was that they adored each other and my main purpose in singing this song for them, was to convey just that.

The wedding day had arrived. After a sleepless night, I had a feeling I was probably not the only one pacing the floor in the middle of the night. I knew however, that everything would be fine. Sally and Michael would pledge their lives to each other, and all the stresses involved in the lead up would fade away, with a simple 'I do'.

What I didn't factor in however, was feeling so nervous. A few nerves are a good thing, they can be used to create energy, heightening a performance in a way that takes the performer beyond themselves.

Too many nerves can squeeze and constrict a throat, stifling the breath so it then becomes a battle of will. When this happens, the music is lost. Nothing can flow. It's like all the parts are not connected. When there's a gap in the workings, the mind is fighting the body, which is fighting the will, which is fighting emotion, and this adds up to a *very* big mess.

The speeches were beautiful and Michael, who rarely said more than a few words at family gatherings, spoke in a way that humbly acknowledged the wonderful impact that Sally had made in his life. He was grateful, he was honest. He was a perfect partner for Sally.

I was happy. My stomach churned. I declined my main course and sang. I watched the two young people I loved dance to the music, and knew in my heart they were blessed with each other.

The music climaxed, the dance floor filled.

Sally smiled at me.

It was done.

Vocal Tea Remedy

This tea is an amazing remedy for any person who uses their voice a great deal.

It can soothe a tired throat and help stop a cold in its tracks, if taken regularly at the first sign of a symptom.

Two to three cups a day can do wonders. It's important to have fresh, good quality ingredients. The quantities given are for a single serve.

Ingredients:
3-4 slices fresh ginger
2-3 star anise
½ lemon juiced and 1 slice
1 teaspoon honey (Manuka preferred)
Boiling water

Taking a Bow

Singing at the wedding was a privilege and it reminded me of many things. It brought back the fundamental basis of what singing meant to me – the sharing of myself.

The giving of my most personal gift.

My voice.

I remembered the day I decided to retire from singing. I was amazed to find that this occasion had the power to shake me up and take me back to the past.

The gown was waiting on the bed. I was showered and ready. I had only to finish touching up makeup, before having a light dinner and driving into the city.

A SONG BIRD

I'd been singing at Crown Casino for over a year and had fallen into the habit of getting there earlier to relax and meet up with a few of the regulars who came to support me.

Casino Productions supplied most of my work, whether as a solo artist or as a vocal arranger for their production arm. I'd just finished doing the scores and backing for a show at Jupiter Casino in Queensland and was looking forward to the performance tonight in the Oak Room.

I was wearing the gold tonight. This was my favourite dress. It was the one extravagance purchased on sale in Paris on our European trip. Steve was running out of patience until I walked out of the dressing room in the glittering gold-crusted halter-neck, and struck a pose.

'However much it costs ... you simply must have it, Poss ... you simply must.' His eyes wide and bright.

There were so many things I loved about Steve. His open honesty and generosity of spirit was yet another on the long list. I'd never had anything like this dress before. We'd only just flown into Paris, and I was nervous, tired and couldn't speak French ... so I started to cry.

It was almost too good to be true, and in some way I held a sense of guilt. Steve whispered, 'I'll divorce you if you don't agree ... so let's just get it together and go!'

The poor saleswomen were slightly baffled as to what was going on. They probably understood 'divorce', but perhaps the pleadings from Steve were mixing messages.

I fumbled for the French dictionary and sniffed away the tears. *'Pardon* ... I'm a singer ... *a chanteuse.'* The two elegant saleswomen looked at each other and smiled. 'The dress ... it is so ... so ... very beautiful ... *beaux ...* ' This was going nowhere and so I stood up straight, took a deep breath and launched into 'Chanson d'Amour'.

The boutique was large, with little booths tucked between the change rooms. The rich heavy curtains were a soft blue and they echoed the soft stripes on the walls, creating a feeling of grandeur and comfort at the same time. This was a place where I could quite comfortably live.

There were two other customers trying on gowns.

Everyone stopped.

Everyone looked.

I laughed at the applause and gave a small bow. 'I'll think about the dress ... thank you so much for allowing me to try it on ... but even on sale it is ... it is ... *trop cher* ... too expensive.'

As I was getting changed, one of the women, the older of the two, came over to the change room and took the dress from the hook.

She motioned me to the counter as I smiled and turned to leave. She dashed from behind and gave me a piece of paper. I looked at the woman in confusion and then looked at the piece of paper. The woman nodded and smiled. *'Cette robe vous appartient, madam.'* I looked at her bewildered.

Where was Steve? Couldn't he wait to get his coffee?

One of the other customers walked towards me in her elegant aqua sequin number. 'She says ... this dress,' as she looked at the gown on the counter being wrapped, 'this dress ... it belongs to you ... madam ... mmm ... they have adjusted the price tag accordingly, so it looks as though it is your lucky day, madam.'

I looked from one woman to the next, unable to believe what had just happened. Once again I wiped the tears from my eyes and followed the woman back to the counter. As I was walking towards the door holding the most precious bag I had ever carried, the same woman said, 'They said you can come and sing to them any time you like, madam.'

I smiled, my joy exploding. I blew a kiss to the two women who had just made me the happiest girl alive. It was at this moment Steve arrived with two coffees and a baguette.

Back to Melbourne

Melbourne's Crown Casino was busier than usual. I had said hello to my regulars and had done the usual vocal warm-up ready for the performance.

Smoking was allowed in most of the gaming rooms and this played havoc with any vocalist, so there were water bottles on hand, just to keep things functioning.

A CURRAWONG SOMERSAULT

The Oak Room was my favourite room. It was large and had a bar, a room behind the small stage to store your things, and the gaming tables were to one side, which allowed a reasonable amount of space for people to sit and drink or rest from gambling.

I worked through my repertoire and the crowd were enjoying themselves. The gold diamantes sparkled as I moved with the melody and I could see the reflections bounce off the walls in front of me. I smiled.

I was wearing Paris.

'Hey Big Spender' was a favourite and was always requested so I slipped into the back room and donned the long black gloves and feather boa. The crowd were starting to clap. The atmosphere was electric and I could sense something.

Something was going to happen. There was the note. It was deep and low. It was now or never. It was held and then I started to slide. To slide a note from chest voice to head voice is tricky and any vocalist will tell you it can be unpredictable. Sometimes it can work and other times …

I took a chance. I slid the note slowly up the scale, way up into the heavens at full force. The feather boa was now reaching for the sky and the breath held strong. I could see the glittering chandelier, the lights flickering stars around the room.

Eyes were wide. Waiting.

Effortlessly and in full control, I reached the high C and

held it. Held it ... held it ... and held ... until ... until I thought I might expire. Mrs Symonds was in front of me and I watched her hands as they floated carefully up the scale, through the haze of smoke.

Higher, higher they soared, her eyes bright and shining, urging me to reach the sky ... and still I held ... I watched her fingers close together, held on ... an eyebrow lift ... a moment more ... the signal clear ... and then ... and then it was done.

The applause was like nothing I had ever experienced at Crown. All the gaming tables had stopped and were clapping. I looked around the whole room, noticing everyone I could. I held them with gratitude. I had stopped, slightly breathless and flushed happy and content, and bowed. I sent a prayer of thanks to Mrs Symonds and once again felt enormously blessed.

The phone call was brief. It was nothing to do with my ability, in fact, if anything ... there was too much of it. I was no longer required to entertain in the Oak Room and was instead directed to the Sports Bar. I didn't know it at the time, but no one had ever interrupted the gambling tables before. This was something that was not to be repeated.

The following week I walked past the Oak Room, on my way to the other venue, poked my head around the corner, curious to see what I had been replaced with. The staff were kind, they always were, they were sorry I was no longer there.

I was grateful for their care.

I understood. These things happen.

The guitarist was sitting on a high stool. He strummed and sang the gentle songs. My heart beat a little faster. There was no one there listening but the gaming tables were busy. I felt sad and deeply sorry for the guitarist and hoped he could find some joy in his playing. You have to be tough to be a muso – you have to have resilience to survive.

So amid the sport blaring from the oversized screens, the punters smoking and drinking, and the call for 'Number 32 to collect their schnitzel and chips' over the loudspeaker system ... I made the decision.

For nearly 20 years I had enjoyed a professional singing career, performing in Adelaide at the Adelaide Casino, the Arts centre and in venues around Australia.

Melbourne had opened up many opportunities including the a cappella group *Vocamotion*, touring in an Elvis tribute show, TV appearances, five-star hotel gigs and co-writing and performing the show *I'll Take Manhattan*, a tribute to the Manhattan Transfer in numerous venues including the George Fairfax Theatre and Mietta's.

Now however,
was
the perfect
time
to retire.

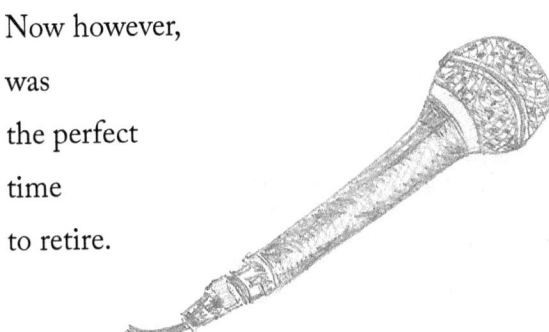

June 2020

On June 12th, tens of thousands of people flooded the streets in cities and towns around Australia and the world. Despite the Australian medical authorities warnings, the recent death of American George Floyd in police custody had inflamed the hearts and minds of people worldwide.

Very little had changed regarding the treatment of Indigenous people in custody since the first Australian Royal Commission, and this latest injustice hit a very deep chord.

Justice versus Virus.

Two very different wars and lives were on the line ... literally. Never was there a more poignant time to highlight the differences. The risks were real. Group gatherings of this scale made social distancing virtually impossible to maintain.

The government and health authorities braced themselves for a second wave of the virus and Steve and I held our breath as we watched the news broadcast.

Would Australia recover from this? Would such a show of unity and strength reap the reward so many hoped to achieve with the protests? Or would the virus be the main beneficiary.

Once again the world was vulnerable.

CHAPTER 22

Open Space

Steve packed the little car and finally we were ready to go. This was the first time we had been anywhere since lockdown, and even the car seemed to sense that this trip would be very good for everyone concerned, its battery included. It didn't take much to fill the boot and in some ways, having such a small car was good incentive to travel light.

In other ways, it caused enormous stress for Steve's creative packing abilities and because of this, the dream of a larger car often dominated conversation whenever we ventured anywhere. I listened, nodded, understood the dilemma he faced, and tried to think of anything *other* than the pain that was starting to dominate my thoughts. Sitting was still the worst position for me. I used icepacks and painkillers to assist, but until things were numb it was hard to concentrate on anything. 'Just relax, Poss ... I'm driving, it's safe ... please don't clutch the door handle to that degree ... you're making me nervous ... relax ... and please stop looking around so much ... just ... relax.'

Some things are easily said and some things are *not* so easily done. I had long given up on the idea of trying to control the back pain that sometimes overwhelmed me, or to hide it from those closest. I'd learnt a great deal about myself over the past six years, and Steve had done his best to support and understand.

He would acknowledge and reassure. He always offered a positive whenever there was any incremental improvement, though currently sitting as I was, in pain that was mine alone, I once again realised he couldn't *possibly* comprehend the battle I was experiencing in that moment.

Relax? Yes indeed my dear ... that would be an amazing thing in itself.

Cost and benefit

This was the equation that I lived by. Sometimes the physical cost of bearing pain completely outweighed the benefit. I knew without hesitation that seeing my family and spending precious time with them, sharing meals and reconnecting after so long, was worth far more than what pain could throw at me. I would cope somehow ... and I knew the benefit would keep me going, like no other drug could. Love could do that. It had power.

Catherine and Bill had invited us to stay the weekend, to help celebrate Catherine's recent birthday. It had been six months since we had seen each other and I couldn't contain my excitement. I missed them. It would just be the four of us and such a treat.

Then the best news arrived, Steve's other sister Marilyn and husband Peter would be joining us for lunch on Sunday. They wouldn't be staying overnight, but would come for lunch between 11 am and 2 pm and we knew this was a massive effort as it was a three-hour drive either way.

The smoked trout, dill, lemon and breads were safely packed in the cool bag, along with a selection of wine and a rhubarb and apple sponge pudding I had made the day before. I knew that Bill would have the necessary accompaniments to finish it off, so opted not to bring ice cream.

The traffic wasn't too bad and we were already halfway there. This warranted a break to get a take-away coffee, stretch legs and change over my icepacks. At this rate we would arrive earlier than expected, and I secretly hoped a visit to the beach would help me regroup before we officially arrived.

A CURRAWONG SOMERSAULT

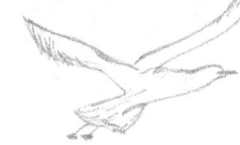

It felt strange looking at the sky and the passing fields, dotted with cattle and sheep. We kept noticing landmarks we knew off by heart, as if it was the first time we had seen them. Being outside felt like a completely new experience.

And there it was. The beach.

I opened my window and a gust of fresh air hit my face. It smelt of the sea. I breathed deeply and felt the cold air fill my lungs, causing a shiver to filter through my body.

'Ah ... at last we made it ... look at the sky, Steve ... have you ever seen anything like it?' Steve smiled broadly and laughed at me. I didn't mind that my hair was flying all around me, getting stuck in my mouth, and giggled with delight as it whipped around my neck. The wind was wild and welcoming, the clouds were flying through the air, fighting for the lead in a race that had no rules.

It had been a long time since we had heard each other laugh and it felt good.

Stepping onto the sand and looking to the horizon brought tears to my eyes. I squinted as the sun pierced through the dark clouds that were gathering along the coastline. It was so beautiful. Steve had already bolted and was heading towards the rock pools that could be seen in low tide. He looked like a young child.

I smiled at his energy, and when he turned and pointed at a fluffy object digging in the sand near him, I laughed out loud. He was an amazing man and after all our years together, it still warmed my heart to see him excited. He had somehow maintained a sense of childhood wonder and often when I least expected it, he would say or do something completely ridiculous and cause my heart to do a backflip in response. I was one lucky woman.

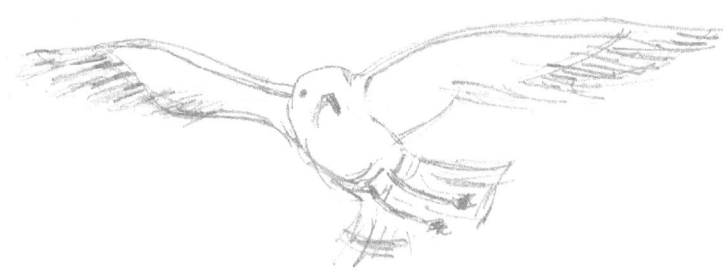

I slowly walked toward him, stopping every few steps to take in the view, not wanting to miss a single detail. My breathing was deep and my eyes stung with the wind. I was cold and I didn't care. There was no one else to be seen. No virus.

The waves glittered, sparkling amid white foam, the roar and crash filled my ears as they came towards me. A large shadow loomed and then it was freezing. Hugging myself I lifted my head to the sky to see a few seagulls trying to fly somewhere and not getting very far. I laughed. Never before had I felt the wonder of space. I opened my arms wide and walked into the wind. 'Oh thank you … thank you for such amazing beauty … it's almost too good to be true.'

I was so grateful to be there. I was so grateful for the expansive horizon and how the sky merged with the shimmering sea. I felt the sea's rhythm inside me as the waves crashed the shore. The wind spoke of freedom and the need to let go.

Tears flowed with the beauty, the salt hit my lips.

I committed it to memory. I knew that I would need this memory in the future and held it … encouraged it … asked it to stay with me. It was at this point that Steve ran up to me, suggesting we go directly to the newsagent and buy a magazine, we were on holiday after all.

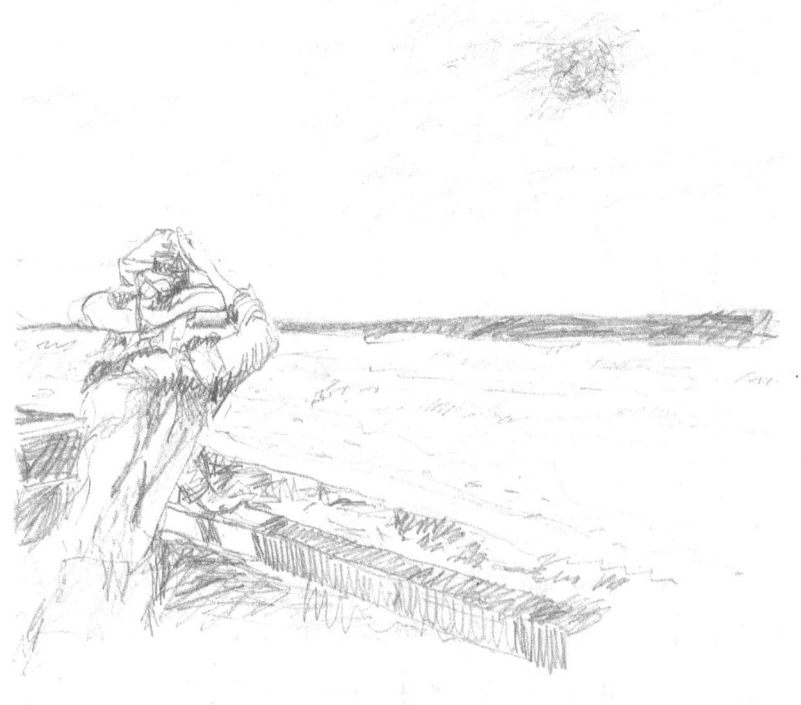

The driveway was spotless, except for a few gum leaves that had fallen and I could see the area on both sides that Catherine and Bill had cleared when they were first in lockdown.

They were determined to get stuck into the garden, while they were forced to look at it and everything looked great. I couldn't believe how much the trees and shrubs had grown. Bright new growth was everywhere to be seen, and the tree house felt sheltered and cocooned in its environment.

It was such a warm welcome. It felt like an eternity since we had last been there and seen each other at Christmas. So much had happened and not happened in that time.

Six Whole Months

It took all of my self-control not to hug them. Somehow, we managed not to embrace due to COVID restrictions.

Staying the required safe distance was instead compensated by enthusiastic laughter, energetic chatter and a flurry of moving things around.

The baggage was deposited in the spare room, the cool bag was safely unloaded to the fridge, with my back icepacks in the freezer, and a cup of tea was already in each person's hand. At last, this felt like home and now we could relax.

The view, as always, beckoned us onto the deck. Weather didn't matter with this view. It was now grey, and the cloud had completely covered the sky, but even so, the wattle birds darted between the branches, and the white galahs shrieked in the distance. Heaven.

I desperately needed to lie down. Catherine and Bill were wonderful at simply knowing instinctively where I was at and it was a relief not having to try and hide my pain from them, I really appreciated that. They had been with me from the start of this pain journey and were one of the few couples who actually understood the challenges associated.

Home is where you can simply be yourself.

Stretching out on the bed I looked out at the trees blowing in the wind. I could hear the rise and fall of conversation in the lounge room above me, a burst of spontaneous laughter, and then a succession of heavy steps clomping around the room. I smiled because these were the sounds of my family and I loved every single one. Sometimes treasure can be found in the simplest of things.

Bill lit the fire. He knew what this would mean to me. I was a fire-a-holic and as my friend Megan would testify, a chronic poker. I had no recollection of when my love of fire began, but I'm sure the old wood oven that my mother cooked on when I was very young probably had something to do with it.

I was allowed to put a log on the fire if very careful and in the height of winter, when the fire had gone out, my mother would put my pyjamas in the oven to warm them up ready for bed. It was such a wonderful feeling jumping into a freezing bed, pulling the covers up around my ears, and feeling the flannelette warm as toast against my body.

There was also the open fire in the lounge room. This was the only form of heating in the family home, other than an electric bar heater that smelt terrible when first switched on.

The crackle of the fire, the coals glowing red, the intensity of heat if you stayed too close, the unexpected spits that a Mallee root could throw, the smoke, the play of shadows bouncing light on the ceiling, the flames licking the wood and the feeling that there was no better place to be, in all the world.

The fire roared and as Bill placed another piece of wood he apologised for the smoke. The wood was a bit damp and amid the coughing and sneezing, we reassured him we didn't care in the slightest. Happiness is to smell of smoke and I was truly happy.

Catherine served her famous Boeuf Bourguignon with all the trimmings. It was delicious and if that wasn't enough, she had made her special pork terrine and put together a platter that could have been a meal in itself. We may never need to eat again! It was wonderful.

What a perfect evening, the company, the meal together and the added bonus that Geelong and Hawthorn were featured for Friday night footy. Everyone settled on the sofas, satisfied and … suitably distanced, eager to enjoy the game. Many times throughout the evening we clinked our wine glasses together, making eye contact, acknowledging and celebrating the special time being shared.

It then dawned on me that I wasn't the *only* one who had missed my family.

Smiling into the flames, I felt warmth flow deeply through my body and once again gave thanks. The virus may have caused enormous stress and uncertainty in all our lives, but it also highlighted without a doubt just who, and what, were most important. This was as clear and bright as the glowing embers flickering before my eyes.

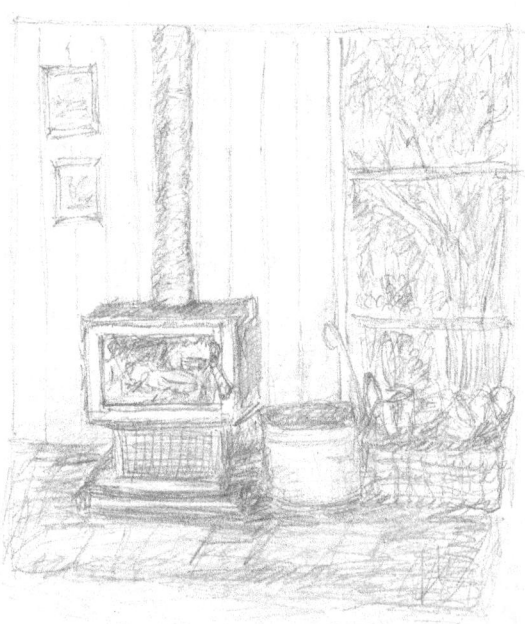

CHAPTER 23

Uncertain Times

The government was issuing statements once again. Not to the same level of intensity seen at the beginning of the pandemic, but often enough to revive the unease that this virus was here to stay for a while, and we had better not become complacent.

There were hotspots flaring up in some of the outer suburbs and many people were queuing for hours to be tested for the virus. Some 20,000 tests were reportedly done in a single day, which stretched pathology groups to their limits.

I had scheduled to open up for business the week after the government restrictions eased for gyms and studios, just to allow time for things to settle. There seemed to be a wait and see what happens scenario to all decisions and each day was the great unknown. I was learning that time would tell all with this virus. Two weeks until opening for business meant I needed to be cautious and respectful of it.

Opening again was going to take a lot of trust on both sides. I knew I was probably erring on the side of obsession in all cleaning practices, but I would also need to trust my clients, because things could unravel very quickly, if they were not diligent.

I wondered whether perhaps I should be tested for the virus prior to reopening? I was thinking it may be a wise thing to do, even though I was well and had no symptoms. So I made enquiries regarding testing sites nearby and how to register.

What I didn't factor in was that every other man, woman, child and dog in the neighbourhood and beyond it had the same idea. I spoke to the security guard overseeing proceedings. 'What time would you suggest I arrive to avoid the queue numbers? This is where I live … so … I can swing by anytime.'

He was tired, he must have answered this question a thousand times a day. He was leaning on the post nearby and was probably in need of a break. He couldn't see my smile behind the mask.

'You're best to get here really early, lady ... and avoid lunchtimes ... sorry can't offer much more than that.'

He then walked up to the last man in line, stood next to him, showed him something on his phone and suggested he come back tomorrow.

I rang my doctor to ask his advice. He could see my point, but said a test probably wasn't necessary, as I had no symptoms and hadn't been in contact with anyone who had been tested.

He did suggest another venue, which was a drive-through testing site, if I wanted to take it further. I was happy not to.

I remembered the bewildered faces. A weird and varied mix of people, all worried and anxious, cold and cautious, spaced and not spaced.

The long line snaked its way around the public building's boundary, zigzagged around the corner and continued halfway down the street.

Then a bizarre thought occurred to me. What a horrible twist of fate it would be if I contracted the virus, while queuing up to be tested for it. The thought sent a shiver through my body.

Turning to leave I walked home briskly, washed my hands thoroughly, and promptly put the kettle on. With cup in hand, I once again felt the enormous relief that being at home could bring.

These were trying times. It started to rain. Looking out the kitchen window I could see the dark clouds gathering over the rooftops and could smell that rain was on its way.

Those poor people in line for testing will be getting drenched.

I thought about the security guard. He wasn't wearing any protective gear and was dealing on the front line. The doctors inside would probably be suitably decked out.

I hoped he would stay safe.

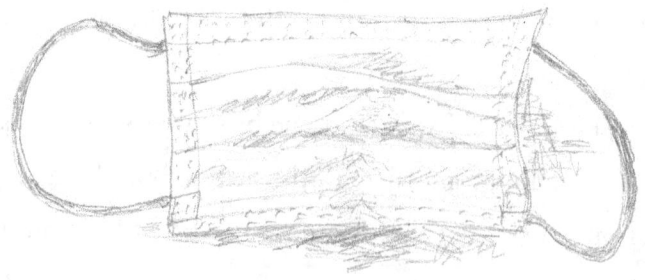

CHAPTER 24

Business Not as Usual

Steve had kindly vacuumed the studio and helped with the intense cleaning in preparation for business commencement. It was the 23rd March of 2020 since I'd been there and all surfaces needed a good scrub. It soon sparkled and smelt of disinfectant. I hoped my clients weren't reminded too much of a hospital setting, so sprayed a few squirts of my favourite perfume in the air.

Moving around the space, it was obvious that the combination of smells was very strange indeed. Steve coughed, spluttered and quickly opened the windows nearby, declaring, 'That scent will definitely not catch on in a hurry.'

He was right, and a few sprays of air freshener were tried next to diffuse the scent confusion.

I was excited to be starting up business again. I'd missed my clients and even though I'd maintained contact with them, it was never the same as dealing face to face.

It was a strange time to begin, as on the 6th of July school holidays were just about to kick in, with many people doing something local to entertain their children over the break.

Even so, I welcomed the opportunity to help anyone who was around and working only a couple of hours a day would help find the new rhythm, which was now focused around major cleaning between client appointments.

It was also ironic opening the business at the same time that Victoria was experiencing the highest daily recorded numbers of the virus.

Yesterday was the highest number, at 44 transmissions. The day before was 41.

These numbers were concerning. The government was still doing a testing blitz for all people affected in outer suburban areas, but even so, the feeling was of unease. I hoped that things could be contained, and contained fast.

Thinking about that reminded me I had better make contact with my brother and sister-in-law. They lived near Hallam, and this suburb was tucked between some of the most high-risk areas. They'd both been able to continue working throughout the pandemic as their jobs were deemed essential services so in some way their routine was unaltered. I needed to make sure they were safe.

> *"Clowns to the left of me, jokers to the right, here I am, stuck in the middle with you"*
> – Stealers Wheel, 1972 (Gerry Rafferty & Joe Egan)

It was becoming impossible to have a conversation. We were now completely surrounded by noise, and looking out the rear bedroom window, I felt I could easily have a chat to the crane driver opposite. It could be a very interesting experience if we learned some sign language skills. I looked down, gasped and wrapped my dressing gown more securely.

Maybe not, and closed the blinds.

A derelict house at the rear of our apartment complex was in the throes of being flattened. Our walls were shaking and the crashing and banging were nothing compared to the vibrations underfoot, kindly directed by Mac or Macca, the crane driver. Only his close friends called him by the latter, and so far I was quite happy to keep things professional. Even though we hadn't formally been introduced, the name seemed to suit him perfectly in my mind.

It was in moments like these that I was so grateful to have enjoyed the freedoms and space of my childhood upbringing in the country. I loved the buzz and vibrancy of city life, but in the confined conditions of lockdown that buzz was now driving me insane. All it took was a smell of fresh air and I could cast myself back to the wide expansive sky filled with flickering stars. How many had I wished upon? Countless dreams made their way to the heavens from our backyard.

A whiff of smoke took me to our family farm when burning off the dry undergrowth meant an opportunity for roasted marshmallows when the embers were glowing bright. Cut grass meant hide and seek in the haystacks or running wild around the dam. Space in all its glory could be accessed when now four walls meant the complete reverse.

Another crane was being erected a block away, in the opposite direction. I could not hear myself think. The song came to mind in a flash and I couldn't help myself. I substituted one word.

'Crane's to the left of me, crane's to the right, here I am, stuck in the middle with you.' I sang at the top of my voice and laughed at the same volume. Steve texted from the other room and I laughed again.

We had started messaging each other when too lazy to literally walk a dozen steps, to the where the other person was situated. Steve had heard something. He thought I had asked him to make us a cup of coffee and I couldn't stop laughing.

The reply was prompt. 'Oh yes please, that would be lovely … you must have read my mind … or something.'

I really must scream more often.

Getting up early for work was a shock to the system. I was so excited to be seeing all my clients again, that the night before was a complete write-off. There had been no sleep, regardless of telling myself how ridiculous I was to be going over everything. Not a great start, as I knew that pain did not respond well to lack of rest. I would simply have to do my best and hope I could get through the morning.

Years before I would have felt disappointed with myself. This way of thinking only pulled me down, adding to the load that pain provides. I wanted to give my best, and I now understood that I would do that regardless of how things felt at the time. I no longer needed to add pressure on myself as I had learnt to trust my ability and awareness in the moment.

To be kinder to myself.

To accept and live with pain instead of fighting it.

Everything was prepared. There were gloves, masks, sanitiser, soap, wipes, paper towel, disinfectant, sprays of every type, a temperature reading device and I should really be a majority shareholder in some of these products by now.

How wonderful it was to see and hear how each client had coped over lockdown. They were in fine form, and most had been diligent and kept their in house exercise routines going, along with walking and stretching. I was so proud of them. Like everyone, they had the choice to either use the time wisely ... or not.

So far, I was encouraged that they were positive and fairly upbeat. Numbers for daily infections were on a steady rise. Yesterday was 77, the highest on record. I reassured them that I would do everything in my power to maintain status quo, and they all marvelled at the way life as we knew it had been turned on its ear.

What touched me more than anything was that it was clear they were also genuinely pleased to see me and keen to bring back some normality to their lives.

Once again, I realised how lucky I was to be working in this field, and just how much each of these people meant to me.

The sun shone briefly through the studio window, and a small rainbow was reflected on the white wall inside.

This was a common occurrence in the height of summer and it seemed unusual for winter to show such a treat. It was a welcome sight however, and cheered my heart. I placed my hand on the wall and watched the colours filter through my fingers. Each colour was clear and yet when I moved ever so slightly, they merged somehow, blending together to create another range of colour. I marvelled at the beauty, the simplicity and the way they moved together. As I drew my hand away the reflection became stronger on the wall. Clear.

VIRUAL ESCAPE LOCKDOWN

Smiling now I remembered my last client, so buoyant and positive amid the fear of what the virus and a chest infection could do to her. An attractive resilient woman, who at 82 years of age battled with limitations, but who *never* allowed them to take over her will or desire to live the best possible life.

Yes, I was privileged to work with such remarkable courage. There wasn't a day that passed without learning something from the wealth of personal experience that my clients brought to my door. The rainbow gleamed, and somehow its splendour spoke of hope.

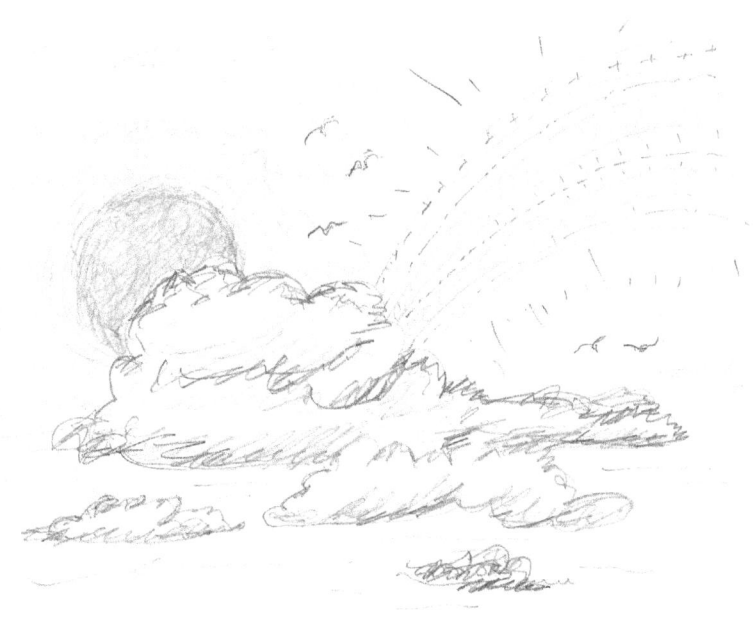

A CURRAWONG SOMERSAULT

CHAPTER 25

Virtual Escape Lockdown

It had been 20 years since Steve and I had been on a decent break. We'd managed a four-week whirlwind tour of Europe, when we'd both been earning reliable incomes, however constant job changes, unemployment and being self-employed had shifted the idea of a holiday firmly down our list. Years rolled into each other, and priorities shifted and changed with the landscape. We were happy where we lived and grateful for what we had, so we found other creative ways to explore the unknown.

I love all things French, so when Rick Stein's Odyssey started a virtual journey by barge on the Canal du Midi, from

Bordeaux to Marseilles, I booked myself first class to join the adventure. There were two sofas in our apartment, so Steve could come along if he so desired. Economy was situated on the floor on a cushion, something I was sure Bitey Boy would have chosen, especially if Chalky was going on the journey.

Both dogs were a touch feisty however, so I wasn't exactly sure how that would pan out.

The cheese platter was ready, the red wine was poured. The music commenced, and we were off. The pace was a bit of a dawdle. Tall, statuesque trees lined the banks and swayed gently in the breeze. It was warm, which was lovely, because winter in Melbourne was becoming dreary. We had just started nibbling our cheese and biscuits, when Rick suggested we stop and take a stroll in a nearby village. I absolutely loved village markets, and so agreed that would be a wonderful idea!

Markets of any description filled me with joy. Food markets in particular set my heart a-flutter and as we all walked around the stalls, I marvelled at the size of the aubergines, the perfectly stacked bunches of pink radishes, and the plump red strawberries begging to be eaten. I hit pause on the TV, and excused myself because I just knew there were some over-ripe strawberries hiding somewhere in the fridge, and started to reshuffle the contents.

'What are you doing, Poss?'

In these situations, Steve's patience evaporated into thin air.

TAKE 2 - PARTIAL LOCKDOWN

I returned with a bountiful bowl of fresh fruit, and in the same amount of time it took to protest, he was settled comfortably with a strawberry in his mouth.

Happiness is good food.

Happiness is sharing it together.

Happiness is sharing it together in the French countryside.

The light was stunning, and there was a glow that seemed to surround everything. A hue, which sparkled on the gentle waves, played with the grasses swaying in the fields, reflected on the swallows that darted through the branches and shone in the eyes of those on board. Everyone was happy.

I smiled as we watched Rick explain the simplicity surrounding a tomato, caper, red onion and goat cheese salad. His cheeks were on fire and we were sure he had started on the wine, well before we had. I secretly hoped he was planning something a little more substantial for lunch, or they would all be very nicely sozzled, before arriving at the next scheduled stop. But then, they weren't driving, so did it really matter after all?

He had read my mind, because the on board cook, who was also the captain, was now in the throes of cleaning up after Rick, and not too happily either. It was quite clearly his kitchen, and he was about to show us all a thing or two about cooking.

This was a dish of fresh prawns and anchovies, shallots and beans. Perfect and simple.

We all retreated to the deck, to give him the space he needed, and to soak in the balmy evening and before we knew it, the time had come to retire and reflect on the wonderful day we had enjoyed. We hit the pillow, happy and satisfied that once again France had not disappointed. We really must travel by barge more often.

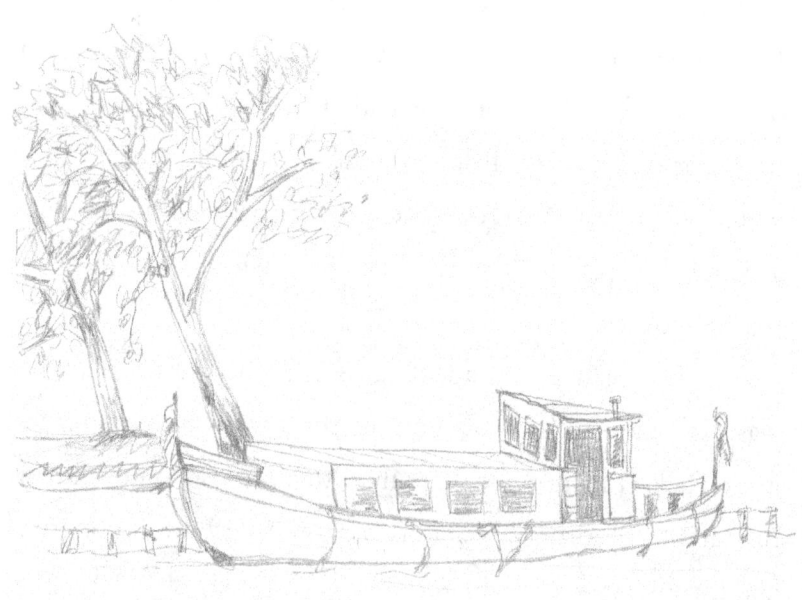

CHAPTER 26

Take 2 – Partial Lockdown

Premier Daniel Andrews was centre stage. Victoria was now at a critical point.

Thirty-six suburbs in Melbourne's north and northwest were to be locked down from the 30th of June 2020, according to their postcodes, for one month. It was hoped that the Stage 3 restrictions would put a stop to the increasing virus cases and help eliminate the spread. Seventy-seven cases were reported yesterday.

All of these suburbs were now known as hotspots.

Oh yes, I had heard that term before, many times.

'We'll just do another nuclear PET scan and locate any

hotspots. It's the best way to track where the inflammation is heading, that way we can treat the affected areas specifically.'

The virus and pain had a few parallels. Both were unpredictable – both got out of control very quickly. The main difference, as far as I could tell, was that the smallest slip up or short cut in dealing with this virus could wipe out any diligence previously done. The result set a roaring fire under it, allowing it to leap and blaze victorious throughout the community. It was very dangerous. One step forward, and 15 steps back to the bunker.

Steve and I were once again baffled at how things had escalated so quickly. There was discussion around the suitability of contract security workers overseeing the travellers in hotel quarantine. There had been alleged breaches. Surely the Australian Defence Force would be best equipped to oversee the affected locations? We hoped it wasn't too late.

School holidays in Victoria had officially commenced and New South Wales issued a very strong warning. They were not happy to see any Victorians whose address matched the postcodes affected.

They were serious. There would be an $11,000 fine and six months jail for anyone who dared. Coincidently, a strange increase in address change applications had been received by the RACV licencing department. I hoped there was no connection and also hoped my community could hold its nerve.

TAKE 2 – PARTIAL LOCKDOWN

Endurance

Any elite athlete will tell you that it takes an enormous amount of determination to reach a desired goal. Some are gifted from the beginning, and fall naturally into the sport that best suits their physique. Others are faced with the added challenge of working with physical attributes that can limit, or a disability that requires a more strategic approach.

I love athletes and admire them. I understand the physical effort required to hone your body into line, and marvel at the enormous variety of elite sports on offer.

Each impose their own unique demands on their bodies, and each need carefully planned care and guidance to achieve peak performance.

The time in preparation.

The need to stay focused.

The commitment to go beyond.

We all start somewhere. Laughing to myself, I remembered the twins taking their first tentative steps, four years ago. Malcolm and Jessica were soon attached to the animated cheers and clapping, which were associated with going beyond the first wobbly steps.

I could remember watching Malcolm manoeuvre around the coffee table, shuffle along the lounge suite, extend an arm to the door frame and slide down the hallway. The whole performance, complete with cheeky grin, was very charming, because he maintained eye contact from beginning to end. This amount of effort needed to be noticed and the funny thing was, that he kept doing it over and over again, until everyone, except him, was completely exhausted.

Such determination and so happy to receive his reward. Before long, the twins were both running uncontrollably down the hallway, there were no gears and certainly no brakes.

It was all or nothing – unbridled abandon. The sheer excitement of being able to move, replaced being plonked in a spot being left to gaze at everything else moving around them.

Now was the time to escape, and finding their feet meant they could do just that, anywhere else was a good place to go and they ran there non-stop!

And then there were scooters. Whoever invented scooters may not have had children, or on second thoughts, it may have been a very cunning plan to lose a few.

'Excuse me, have you seen a couple of kids go by? A small boy with corduroy pants and a little blond girl in a pink tutu? They were here a minute ago … and then all of a sudden …'

What started with such effort had somehow been replaced with wild adventure. The focus wasn't so much on getting their bodies to *cooperate* to do something, but more about the *destination* they were headed. Going somewhere quickly was now the priority and their bodies simply went along for the ride.

Never before had Steve and I realised the effort involved in raising children. It was non-stop. We felt privileged to be involved in the twins' small world, and marvelled at how so much of their early development seemed instinctive. They were becoming little people.

Many theories abound regarding whether we are pre-programmed or destined to become who we are. I often wondered about this and also how I came to be part of my family unit.

I had a sense I might have been accidentally misplaced, and a few times I considered checking the hospital birth records. Perhaps there had been an unusual spike in births for October? Maybe the January school holidays had been especially pleasant, and as a result many babies entered the world nine months later?

I knew I was a surprise pregnancy. The mind boggled.

Accidents can happen ... one baby ... another baby ... who knows ... there may have been a switch.

It did amuse me. The idea that some other family, somewhere, were still trying to figure out why their child *didn't* have a musical, creative bone in her body.

A CURRAWONG SOMERSAULT

CHAPTER 27

Stamina

Both Steve and I had just about had it! We were starting to feel that if we heard 'we're all in this together' one more time … we may not be responsible for our actions.

The message had worked a treat, in the early stages of the pandemic when everyone was in lockdown. The idea that all people, both here and around the world, were united in trying to stop the virus spreading and killing helped reassure the fears and uncertainties of the time.

Everyone was in lockdown.

Everyone who wasn't a hoarder, was looking for toilet paper.

Everyone whose business had been shutdown, was worried.

Everyone missed their family.

Everyone missed their friends.

Everyone felt lost.

Everyone felt vulnerable.

We were in it together. There were those who decided they were more important than others. There were those who put their own needs above everyone else's. Some people disregarded the guidelines and did their own thing. Others didn't care.

We were given clear guidance, with a sense of urgency to do the right thing, not only for our own safety, but to protect the lives of others. It was a blatantly clear message. If we were not responsible, we would be literally killing the vulnerable.

We were all getting tired and if Steve and I were feeling this way, then there were probably others who were also starting to feel the load caused by this virus.

There were those who worked tirelessly to support the vulnerable. There were those who kept turning up to face the medical demands. Some people delivered food to communities they'd never met, others sacrificed their own health to save lives.

The virus was the same. Something else had changed.

The Weekend

The silence was such a relief. Sunday morning was the only day of the week that all the building works took a break, and I had been hanging out for this. Reluctantly opening my eyes I slowly turned to look at the clock. Perfect.

It was early, so I turned over, pulled the covers around my ears and settled down to continue the dream.

Daydreaming in bed was a wonderful thing, especially when it was quiet. And then a 'squawk ... whah ... whah ... whaaaaah!'

Gosh, that little girl next door was hungry! She was now six weeks old and was often seen as a wobbly head, tucked into her mother's sling as she went about her business.

It was a reassuring routine in some ways; a few squawks, some soothing words, a random bark from Dudley, a few more squawks and then silence, as the little family settled once again.

I sighed. And then a crow.

Crows have innate instinct. They are large. They are black. They are heavy and loud, and they know how to use these attributes. They are attracted to a tin roof. Their preference is a flat tin roof. They particularly like flat tin roofs with skylights. I pulled the covers over my head. 'It's Sunday for goodness sake, give me a break!'

Their sole purpose in life was to wake up anyone who may have just drifted off to sleep.

Steve snored a little louder. I sighed again. Oh well, there's always next Sunday. Quietly getting up, I made a cup of tea and sat downstairs for a while, determined to greet the day in a relaxed manner.

It was grey. There was a forecast for rain and possible hail.

We would probably go to the market.

Maybe not, if there was hail.

I pulled the woollen throw over my legs and looked at the courtyard oasis. Winter held very little colour. There was one little marigold poking its head through the parsley. What a cheery little flower. I refilled my cup and took one upstairs for Steve. Chances are he'd sleep for another few hours so I crept back into bed, snuggled up to him and tried to resume the interrupted daydream.

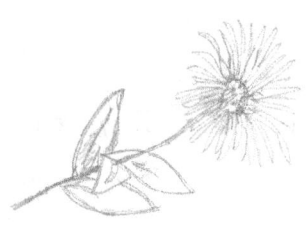

"In Freudian psychology and psychoanalysis, the reality principle, is the ability of the mind to assess the reality of the external world, and to act upon it, accordingly, as opposed to acting on the pleasure principle."

– Based on Sigmund Freud's Reality Principal, 1896

Daydreaming had its place. Sometimes I could focus so intently on something that I'd find myself in a completely different environment. Imagining had the power to do that.

I loved nothing better than to pore over design magazines and soak up the clever ideas.

The best part was then to play with them in my mind, add this, delete that, and create my own version, messing around until there was no resemblance to the original at all.

This could go on for hours. I had designed and decorated so many homes in my imagination that the process of putting things together felt natural and fun. It would begin like this – I could sit or lie in a little courtyard, flanked with either wisteria or elm trees.

I'd gaze into the bird bath which was adapted from an old cedar wine barrel or huge copper cooking pot and notice the reflections dance on the wall of sliding glass or wooden bi-fold doors nearby.

Picking up the fallen leaves, I considered whether replacing the scoria pebbles lying underfoot with grey slate paving would be a better option?

It would reduce the noise level when walking around outside, and would certainly make cleaning up the leaves much easier. A high hedge may be worth consideration?

I could simply transplant the trees and place them behind the courtyard drystone wall and this would create a sense of height, with the hedge giving symmetry.

Perfect.

The options were endless and each simple change created an entirely different feel. One thing affected the next, which in turn affected what was next to that, which then meant the whole area was gradually morphing into something completely different.

It was fascinating.

The relationship of things. It wasn't just where they were placed, but whether they needed to be there at all. Ideas would often be flowing nicely, and then all of a sudden they would stop.

Something wasn't right.

What is going on here? The colours work, there's a flow to the first room into the living area ... the light and shade are complementary to the furnishings ... but something's not right ... something ... feels ... off kilter.

In my mind, I moved around the area, surveying it from different angles. I went outside and looked in. I ventured down the entry hallway and looked back.

I walked slowly around the main living area and stopped to observe. I even managed to attach myself to the ceiling and look down.

STAGE 3 – MELBOURNE LOCKDOWN

It was in this position I saw it at once. Ah-hah! There's too many chairs in relation to walkway space and this ... had stopped the flow, reducing the walkway ... and also stopping the eye travelling to the main courtyard and beyond.

With balance restored, there was once again a sense of calm. A sigh, that felt better.

It was finding the feel of it that appealed the most. To explore space, style, colour and design was an added bonus, in the quest of the feel. In a strange way, it was like the relationship between music and melody.

It could affect the listener in so many varied ways, with each person responding differently, even though it was the same piece of music.

One person could be overwhelmed by emotion and brought to tears, another could be given a sense of strength and reassurance. It was a mystery.

Time and again, I watched the series *Escape to the Country*, journeying with the city dwellers in the hunt for their dream home nestled in the English countryside.

The poor presenter was often driven to distraction when a couple was shown home after home, each of them meeting the criteria they had asked for, only to hear 'Something's not quite right. We'll know it as soon as we set foot inside ... we can't explain it, there's something missing'.

There were other times when couples were brought to tears, as soon as they walked inside, they'd finally found exactly what they were looking for, it spoke to them somehow.

There was a power beyond themselves, that touched them deeply.

The dream, it had come true.

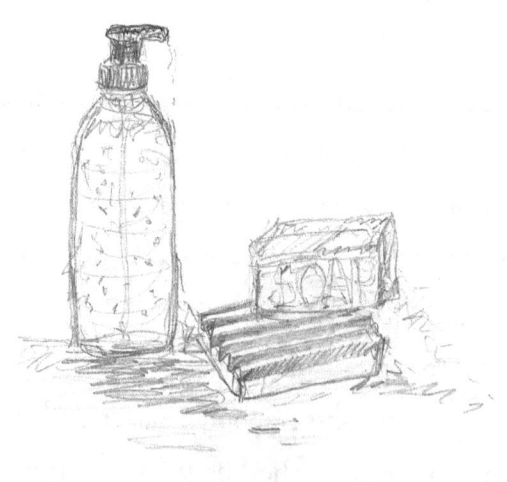

CHAPTER 28

Stage 3 – Melbourne Lockdown

Victoria was out of control. The virus had taken hold and 197 new cases had been reported.

Wednesday 8th July 2020 the borders had been closed to Victoria and once again the state was to recommence the stringent lockdown rules we had started with in March 2020.

I slumped back onto the chair. My clients had started sending messages. 'Are you still working? What was going to happen?' I had officially worked six days since restrictions were eased. It was a rollercoaster and once again we were off and racing – nowhere.

It was sad going back to the studio, packing up again and turning off the power. Cost saving was high on the list of priorities, and we were working to a very strict budget. We had been through hard times before and had learnt how to scrimp and save.

Juggling finances was a challenge, but we were determined not to forfeit our home this time around. The last recession in 1990 had done just that. We had worked two shifts, four jobs between us, just trying to hold onto our gorgeous little cottage in Adelaide. Interest rates that had commenced at 8% spiralled to a whopping 19%, and because of this, we soon owed more than what we were capable of paying. Tough times indeed.

Selling and moving to Melbourne was a fresh start and a chance to put the heartache and disappointment behind us. This valuable lesson was a reminder to *never* take for granted anything we had worked so hard for.

The unpredictable, is just that. Life seems to be always in the throes of change. We take one step after the other, in the hope that we will end up somewhere, working hard to earn a dollar, so that there is food on the table and a roof overhead. Those with children have the added stress of providing for them. It's not new, the centuries have repeated the same. I scanned my phone and responded to my clients. We would all have to hold on, we were all travelling somewhere ... but the destination was completely unknown.

STAGE 3 – MELBOURNE LOCKDOWN

Can you wash away your fingerprints?

I was beginning to wonder whether perhaps it was possible because I'd lost count of the number of times my phone didn't recognise my thumb print to gain access. Phones are pretty smart these days, perhaps it had hooked into my emotional state and thought I needed a rest from it.

Possible, and quite considerate, if so.

The sun was shining and this was the best part of the day. It was a welcome friend, and somehow made the idea that there was a dangerous virus lurking around seem ludicrous.

Opening the rear courtyard doors brought a wonderful surprise. The cranes were taking a momentary break and so I could hear the normal sounds of life. A couple of cars went by, a distant horn, a light plane was passing overhead, and the rattling of a tram seemed to speed up some distance away. The plane returned. It was unusual to see and hear a plane. *That was different, unusual ... different ... oh no ... not Kath and Kim filling my thoughts ... this was not a good sign ... and still another six weeks to go!* I listened, and listened. Not one single bird to be heard. Not one, not even a crow.

And then the plane returned again. It had probably frightened all the birdlife away – they thought it was a massive silver bird and moved on to the next suburb.

I could hear Steve mid-conversation, he was animated and enthusiastic. Gosh I was grateful that he had a few bits and pieces workwise, as it would be a nightmare if we were both wandering around the apartment, looking at what to do next. I messaged him ... Coffee?

This was one of the simplest pleasures in life and at the moment it was our highlight, and always guaranteed a sense of happiness. The smell, the sound, the way Steve became very Italian in his barista movements and explanations.

It was wonderful. We both looked at the dwindling supply of Anzac biscuits in the jar. Had we really eaten the last batch already? Steve shrugged. If that was the worst of our habits in lockdown, then so be it. I knew exactly what I needed to do tomorrow.

Vertical Ships

The thought brought a shiver through my body and made me feel sick. The memory of what happened on the *Ruby Princess* was still quite fresh and something I hoped would not be repeated. There were nine public housing towers in North Melbourne and Flemington placed into lockdown.

Police, nurses and healthcare workers were monitoring the buildings and food was being brought in to help the residents, who had no time to prepare for the five-day lockdown. The idea was to try and contain the virus spread.

Quickly and efficiently.

Would it contain or would it inflame?

STAGE 3 - MELBOURNE LOCKDOWN

Many people complained that they knew nothing about what was happening and police were left to sort out the confusion. Some received food parcels, others didn't, some received out of date foodstuffs, others couldn't eat what was provided because of religious beliefs.

Once again, the government had acted quickly ... yes ... but efficiently? Things were complicated.

We couldn't imagine how the government was able to juggle so many variances. The situation was changing constantly, and by the time something was implemented it was deemed out of date and a new plan was required, and quickly.

We were starting to feel the drag of this situation on ourselves, even though we were just a small cog in a very large wheel.

I worried for the leaders and the enormous weight they must be under: the responsibility they must shoulder. The sleepless nights they must endure, and the stress they felt which filtered through to their families. The pressure of making the right decision at the right time and having to front up every day and deliver news that no one wanted to hear.

The unknown.

Thinking about this reminded me that I must keep my eyes and ears open, and stay alert to what was happening around us. There may be other ways that I could help, apart from just staying at home.

I couldn't bring myself to go to the supermarket because the latest news coverage had shown row after row of empty aisles. I couldn't believe my eyes, once again products had been stripped from the shelves, and rations were again in place for some items, toilet paper included.

Seeing the same panic buying routine made me feel sad. Have we learnt nothing?

Human nature – "The natural ways of behaving that most people share"
– *Cambridge University Dictionary*

A huge sigh escaped as I wondered just how long it would take for this behaviour to run its course.

The inconvenience was irritating, but more importantly, it was the general public I was concerned about. They must be living in a bubble of fear if they haven't realised that produce was still available and would be gradually restocked. They needed reassurance. They needed to feel safe. They needed something tangible.

Having a cupboard full of toilet paper somehow filled that deep, dark void. I wanted to cry. These were my people. I hated the thought that such mundane items were providing what humankind should be sharing naturally. Love. Care.

Rummaging through my bag I found $20 in the sleeve of my wallet. It had been hiding, waiting and I knew exactly what needed to be done. The market called. It was Tuesday, and so

STAGE 3 – MELBOURNE LOCKDOWN

the foot traffic would be less. I'd wear a mask, in case others felt unsafe. We needed a baguette to go with the soup planned for dinner, and so I brought along the hessian bag.

The man was often at the entry of the market. He was bright and cheerful and always asked the same questions, giving a smile, when time and again people declined his offer.

'Have you read the latest issue? There's great stories and articles … do you know the Big Issue?'

Making eye contact. 'Thanks mate, don't worry I'll see you on the way back.' I sanitised at the entry, lined up at the French bakery, purchased the last baguette on offer, and promptly returned to the man out the front.

When I handed over the note, he became flustered and started shuffling all the magazines, explaining every article that might be of interest. I listened and thanked him for being so thoughtful. While listening I wondered whether I should decline and let him sell on the extra copies, but as he enthusiastically continued I realised something important.

He didn't want a handout or what might be interpreted as pity; he was supplying a service and giving important information for a fee. He was so grateful and gave me too many issues. I accepted gracefully and thanked him for his time and explanation.

'I'll enjoy reading these … thanks so much … and will see you again when next at the market!' Some people are far too kind, and I had just met one of the best.

Red Capsicum and Lentil Soup

Ingredients:

1 can organic lentils (drained)

1 can chopped tomatoes

1 large red capsicum (roughly chopped)

2 large carrots (sliced on angles)

1 large brown onion (roughly chopped)

2 cloves garlic (finely chopped)

1 cup hot stock (chicken or vegetable)

1 cup white wine

10-12 sliced green olives

1 dollop tomato paste

Zest of 1 lemon

Herbs – dried chilli flakes (pinch), oregano, marjoram, basil (½ teaspoon each)

LOCKDOWN BIRTHDAY JULY 2020

Method:

In a large saucepan, fry onion, garlic and chilli flakes in a little olive oil for 1 minute.

Add chopped capsicum and fry for a couple of minutes, stirring continually.

Add dried herbs and stir.

Add drained lentils and stir.

Combine hot stock and white wine, then add to the saucepan.

Add lemon zest, sliced carrots, tin diced tomatoes, sliced olives and a dollop of tomato paste.

Stir to combine and check liquid level. You may need to add a little hot water, depending on the size of your saucepan.

Simmer 40 minutes on medium heat.

Check often and skim off any scum that may be on top.

Add another pinch of herbs if you like a more intense flavour. Perfect served with a baguette.

A CURRAWONG SOMERSAULT

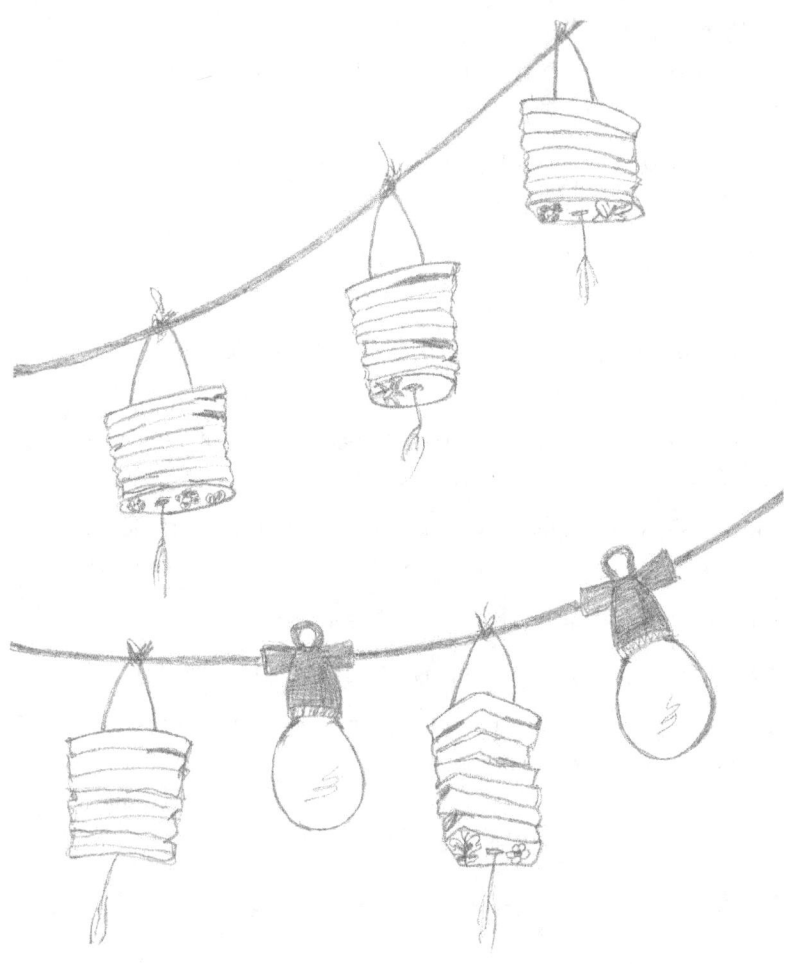

CHAPTER 29

Lockdown Birthday July 2020

A couple of weeks had passed since I'd broached the subject. 'If you could have any cake or dessert you like ... what would you choose?' It was almost impossible trying to surprise Steve.

He had a knack of finding out proceedings. He had a cunning way of seemingly being oblivious to the whispers or conversations in another room, when all the while he was piecing together the hints, elusive looks or indifference, that meant something was going on.

Last year had been enormous because Steve had turned a wonderful age. It was something he wasn't keen to come to terms with, and this avoidance was the main motivation for me to spoil him rotten. Every year was worth celebrating, but this one was not going to slip into space without a bit of fun attached to it. It'd been years since we'd had a good party, a holiday, or anything of note, so this was a great excuse. It was 12 months in the making. The list of friends and family needed advance notice, as many needed to travel interstate or overseas to attend. Babysitters, accommodation and all things associated needed time to organise and then the fun began.

I needed to design the invitations, book the venue and think about its decoration, discuss the menu and logistics, and make numerous lists and time lines, so that everything ran smoothly. What a juggle. Steve was unpredictable. One day he would be going into the city to attend a meeting for a few hours, another day he would be home all day. I had to be careful.

'Any plans as to your day tomorrow?' I'd ask casually. This question was wearing thin and I knew ... he knew ... I was up to something.

It was a race to use the computer upstairs and print out anything needed and I'd often find myself in the throes of printing some photos for a feature wall display, and then hear the front door key rattle the lock.

Then it was a major panic. I'd scramble to gather everything together, turn off the printer, throw things into the cupboard, and as a decoy, flush the toilet just as he casually walked up

LOCKDOWN BIRTHDAY JULY 2020

the stairs. It was wearing – it was wearing me down. It was such a good idea at the time, I only hoped I had the stamina to see it through.

Mary and Paul were flying in from Sydney on the morning of the party and staying overnight.

Paul was to take Steve for copious amounts of coffee mid-afternoon, which would then allow Mary and I to fly into action. We needed to collect the balloons and attach them to the stairwell in the apartment amid a flurry of Chinese lanterns, arrange the flowers ordered from the market, and then deliver them in vases to the venue around the corner. The pizza restaurant was a favourite of ours, so I knew Steve would enjoy what was on offer there and the rear function room was the perfect venue.

There were olive trees flanking the bench seats on one side, and a long table with chairs on the other. Everything sat snuggly under a glass roof, with hanging party lights strung up between the trees. The ambience was lovely at night and the most wonderful thing of all was the large wood fire near the entry, which would add to that feel and also keep everyone warm. Showers were forecast and Melbourne was freezing. Please let the weather hold.

Megan had arrived to assist, and so I left her with Mary, so I could go to the venue and commence the preparation. Time I knew … would go nowhere … very fast.

There was a delay. The previous booking had not yet left and this had bumped out the preparation.

I waited. With only an hour until guests were to arrive, I was starting to worry.

The phone rang. Sally and Michael were just dropping off the twins. 'Did I need any help setting up?' I could have cried. Once again, Sally had come to the rescue and not only was she bringing the croquembouche which was to be the dessert, served with strawberries and cream, but also her very tall husband, who would be perfect to put up the photo display wall on one side of the venue.

I gave a quick prayer of thanks, arranged the flowers, put out the personalised placemats, cutlery, seating guide and gave directions to the staff who were assisting for the evening. Then Mary arrived and helped Sally hang the Chinese lanterns between each of the lights. My main thought now was whether I would make it through the night.

The back pain was becoming unbearable, but this night was one I needed to manage. I went to my bag to retrieve the last icepacks. A trip to the ladies put them in place along with an additional dose of painkillers. I could do nothing more and stopped for a moment looking into the fire.

This is not about me, please help me get through this for Steve's sake and … everyone … he deserves it … please help me … get through.

LOCKDOWN BIRTHDAY JULY 2020

An Enormous Success

Sometimes strength can come from nowhere. I looked at Steve while thanking our guests for travelling from far and wide, to share such a special time together. He was in his element, surrounded by his closest friends and family. History, and the stories it held were shared amid laughter and food and the fire glowed red, along with the flush of pride that I felt for the man who had shared so much of my life.

This would stay with us for a very long time. A few impromptu speeches highlighted the respect Steve held among those closest to him, and as I made my way around the group, it was clear that he was loved for exactly who he was. What a perfect night.

The last glass of champagne meant that the clean-up was to begin and this little songbird was ready for bed. It had been years since I had been up so late. Quite a strange thought when most of my singing life I'd been a night owl. My how things had changed.

As everyone hugged and said their goodbyes, it was agreed that getting older had its merits after all.

Steve, of course, was now keen to share that 'I knew exactly what was going on … however … there were a few surprises.'

The balloons greeted us at the apartment as shoes and tight clothing were replaced with anything more comfortable.

The interstate travellers, Mary, Paul, Marian and Mark, joined us to reflect on the evening and share the highlights that meant something to them. What wonderful friends.

Steve was now wearing the woollen vest that Mary and Paul had given him ... as a joke and this seemed to match perfectly the knee high ugg boots from Megan.

Photos were shared, laughter exploded. This was one night when the young neighbours would wonder when the festivities would end. Not bad for the oldies next door!

Sour Cherry Slice with Ricotta Honey Cream
Steve had finally chosen from the enormous list of cake and dessert that he loved. Had I really cooked so many different desserts?

It was decided. Sour cherry slice with ricotta honey cream was what he would love for his birthday dinner.

Never in a million years could one year be so different to the last and we marvelled at the fact we'd enjoyed such an event last year. It seemed like a world away, almost a blur.

This year would be the complete reverse.

Lockdown birthday.

Steve's birthday had arrived and in so many ways he was still the young boy who waited in anticipation for his special day. I found this so endearing that I couldn't help trying to create something to match his excitement level.

LOCKDOWN BIRTHDAY JULY 2020

Quietly rolling over I looked at him. He was dozing, so I just looked for a while.

He was still the handsome man I'd married many years before; the high forehead, deep-set eyes, perfect eyebrows, well-proportioned nose and very kissable full lips.

The years had been kind to him. He had grown into himself, and even though the hair was not as wild and wonderful, there was still enough to run my fingers through.

I started with a whisper. 'Happy birthday to you ... happy birthday to you ... happy birthday dear Ste-eve, happy birthday to you.' Propping myself up on an elbow I waited. There was no response, the breath was even. I waited. Two could play this game. I repeated the refrain, but this time the whisper was slightly different. The timing was weirdly syncopated with accents on different words. No response, again I waited.

He was testing me out. I knew his tactics, I was good with endurance and waited.

Slowly now I slumped onto my back. I knew exactly what to do, and quietly snuck out of bed and tiptoed downstairs. I switched on the kettle and while that was heating up, went to the secret hiding place and retrieved the three gifts that were stored. I was sure he wouldn't hear that.

The tea was presented on a tray with a selection of his favourite biscuits. I'd been cooking the extra things in between the usual soups and meals, and storing them in weird and wonderful places, so he wouldn't find them prior to the day. The spirit of Bitey Boy had a very sneaky side to him and it took cunning to match it.

Placing the tray next to the bed, I looked down and smiled. He hadn't moved, but I could see his eyes were trying to stay shut and I knew he would be curious, so waited.

I stood next to the bed and then gently placed a present on his tummy. It was a reasonable size and it amused me watching it rise and fall with his breath. Two minutes. He slowly opened his eyes to see my smiling face. 'Oh there you are.'

And launched into a much more vigorous funk version of the song, complete with arm movements and head flicks. The hips and back were not up to getting involved at this hour of the morning.

He stretched and yawned, taking his time to emphasise the moment, as if this was just a usual occurrence and something that happened every day. I waited, but was starting to think that a dressing gown may have been a good idea as it was cold and I couldn't feel my feet.

The movement surprised me and caught me off guard. In a swoop he had moved the present off his tummy and dragged me to the bed. I squealed. He laughed.

He wrapped me up and said, 'So where's my present?' There was nothing to say after that. All I knew was that he had won ... and he was a very ... spoilt ... boy indeed.

LOCKDOWN BIRTHDAY JULY 2020

More Sour Cherry Slice?

The cherry slice was a major success and it was celebrated at lunch, mid-afternoon coffee, and then as dessert for the evening meal. I'd forgotten about this recipe and was glad it was the one that Steve requested. The idea of indulging in sponge cake all day long would have been a bit of a challenge, especially as there needed to be stomach room for dinner.

The table was set. I loved dressing a table, and did this after lunch so that there was time to admire it, and no rush to get things together before dinner.

Our dining table is a solid wooden door. It has legs that match the same wood and is incredibly heavy. If you look closely, you can make out where the door knob has been filled and stained, and the surface undulates, making it sometimes a challenge for wine glasses with fine bases.

The removalists who struggled getting it into the apartment gasped, 'I've never seen anything like it … that's a decent piece of wood there … that is … [puff, puff] … don't go getting rid of that one … in a hurry'.

I love it. It has moved with us for years and sometimes it is enough to just put cork tiles on top, and simply show its uniqueness and other times you would never know it was there.

For Steve's birthday, I had wrapped the table. I'd done this once before for Christmas, using rolls of holly inspired paper, and then covered it with clear cellophane to protect the

Christmas paper from spillage, making it look like a very big present, with real holly leaves scooped at both ends and ribbons wrapping up the whole thing.

It was birthday paper this time, with navy blue and gold stripes. I hadn't factored in the difficulty of working with stripes, but eventually it came together, amid some colourful muttering under my breath. Candles, foliage at different heights, lime green plates and bowls, crystal glasses and a centrepiece of fruit and dried fruit, which sat high on some paper-covered books.

What fun. We both dressed for the occasion, and as the music swayed in the background, we enjoyed the spatchcock stuffed with orange, pistachio and prunes, the baby potatoes and beans, then finished off what was left of the cherry slice. We would never need to eat again. 'Cheers to you my dear … so good of you to have another birthday!'

Three Days Later

Steve had some work to finish off and I felt that if I didn't get outside soon, I might just implode. The recent birthday dinner had been wonderful, however the extra cooking and eating had made me feel sluggish and like a blob.

The heater was on, causing a dreamy sleepiness that only strengthened the feeling that blobbiness was taking over my body … I needed to move.

The sun was shining, so that was a positive.

LOCKDOWN BIRTHDAY JULY 2020

Opening the front door brought with it a huge gust of wind.

Promptly shutting that, I went upstairs for some warmer reinforcements.

Coat, woollen cap, gloves and scarf. Done.

Face mask, just in case. Done.

I hadn't ventured outside for a few days, as lockdown was something that both Steve and I took very seriously.

This was a treat.

Walking onto the street, I noticed the lack of cars and felt that was good. Walking briskly against the wind, I made my way to the end of the street, crossed the road at the school, and followed the sun down the side street. It was great to see the blue sky. I noted the blue and white Greek house, the ramshackle house on the corner, and noticed wattle trees about to burst into flower. They were a bit early; perhaps the sunshine had confused them.

Making my way around the corner, I turned right to walk across the overpass. It was from this vantage point that you could see the vastness of the sky and gain a sense of space. There were white clouds, spreading the sky like freshly washed sheets on one side, and the other was a simple blue. Leaning against the bridge the sun soaked through the first layer of clothing. Beautiful.

It was quiet and memories of the first lockdown filled my mind. No one was really prepared for what lockdown meant.

It was strange and unknown.

There was fear. I breathed deeply and took in the sky.

The warmth, along with the moment, calmed my mind, and I could feel my body relax.

A couple were walking towards me. They were close together, so they must live together.

I decided to cross the road and give them right of way. They nodded. They may have smiled it was hard to tell, they were wearing masks. I waved and smiled into my own mask.

Making my way down the street, I turned left and walked on the sunny side. The sun was illusive between the bursts of cloud, but I was determined to follow it. Zigzagging and weaving, I went down some streets, around others, and then found myself a few blocks away in unfamiliar territory. There were more high-rise buildings situated here, with a few red-brick houses dispersed between them. Hanging baskets filled with red geraniums featured from the front verandas, and scraggly tomato plants battled to show themselves over the fence line.

There was a figure some way in front of me. In fact, it was the conversation that was heard before anything else. 'Have you been? Not worth it … nothing …' as he held the empty plastic bag out in front of him. The arms stayed out, as he waved it around in the air, trying to make very clear that he had not been successful.

As I approached, I saw the woman across the road that he was addressing.

She was leaning over her red-brick fence and responded just as enthusiastically, but in what appeared to be another language. They understood each other. She was totally Greek, and he was a combination of the same, with some English and slang thrown in for good measure.

'What can you do? Supermarket empty … what can you do?'

I noticed his old brown woollen jumper, too short from too many hot washes the wide pants that flapped around his ankles exposing short socks, and the sports cap that was the only thing that seemingly hadn't shrunk. They were on the same side of the road now.

The woman, who sported a green apron and fluffy pink slippers, was now across the road and giving some reassurance? No … maybe support? … No … I wasn't exactly sure what she was giving, but I edged my way close to the curb to give them a wide berth. The theatrical arms in particular needed the space, forget the 1.5 metres.

They didn't see me so I slipped across the road and down the next small street. Still hearing the discussion, I marvelled at the cultural diversity of our neighbourhood. Observing this exchange had transported me somewhere else … Greece – in my own backyard. I hoped he had better luck tomorrow.

Sour Cherry Slice with Ricotta Honey Cream

Ingredients:

1 cup caster sugar

2 eggs

¼ cup Marsala wine

1 cup plain flour

1 teaspoon baking powder

½ teaspoon salt

1 cup chopped walnuts

1 tin drained cherries (no pips)

Honey cream

200 g fresh ricotta

⅓ cup honey

Method:

Preheat oven to 180°C (160°C fan forced) and line base of a rectangular tray with baking paper.

Place sugar, eggs and Marsala wine in a bowl. Use an electric mixer and beat 5 minutes until slightly thickened and lighter in colour.

In a large bowl, combine flour, baking powder, salt and walnuts. Add egg mixture and fold gently until evenly mixed.

Gently fold in cherries last.

Pour into prepared tin and bake 45 minutes to 1 hour or until just golden and the centre springs back.

Cool in tin for 5 minutes, then turn onto a wire rack to cool.

In a medium size bowl, whisk ricotta and honey until light and creamy.

Serve in squares, sprinkled with icing sugar and a dollop of honey ricotta.

CHAPTER 30

Numbers Say It All

Lockdown for Victoria happened in the nick of time. Cases of the virus were escalating, with 288 newly transmitted cases yesterday. This was more than a wave. These numbers were far greater than at the beginning of the pandemic, so the government recommended that masks should be worn whenever possible, in addition to the strict cleaning and distancing routine already in place.

Victoria had 3,379 cases and had recorded 22 deaths on the 10th of July 2020.

Australia as a whole had tallied 9,359 cases and 106 deaths. Many recoveries had been made, but shadows lurked behind the numbers and I knew that the risk for the vulnerable increased enormously with each jump in transmissions. Each of these numbers represented a person and no one wanted to die at the hand of this virus.

I pulled the covers over my head. Was July usually this cold? Stupid question it's winter remember. Bed socks may be a good idea tomorrow night, and promptly turned over.

I needed a break from the news.

It was starting to affect me deeply.

America was on a downward spiral. They had recorded 3,291,786 cases and lost 136,000 people to the virus. President Donald Trump was under the illusion that they had contained the virus, and was issuing statements that made no sense. As a result, the numbers exploded.

This virus was capable of wiping out entire populations.

The sheer weight of the numbers hit me extremely hard.

I cocooned myself by curling up into a ball. My mind was blank. No amount of wishing was going to make anything different for those poor people. I hoped someone would rise up and present some common sense, before the whole American nation was destroyed. I wept.

The tears were for those people whose lives had been cut short. The families, who were unable to be there when their loved ones needed them most. The frustration of the medical staff, who had done everything they possibly could.

"Desperate times call for desperate measures"
– Hippocrates, 460BC

I sat up in bed. This was going nowhere ... fast. I looked out the window and watched the rain trickle down the sill. It was at that moment the annoying dripping commenced to hit the metal window pane, reverberating through the wall, directly to my right eardrum.

I watched and listened. No amount of silicone or creative theory had solved that one.

It seemed that water was not easily tamed and the drips continued triumphantly. I sighed, I needed to get a grip.

Looking out the window I saw a bird flying high into the sky. I craned my neck to hold the image as it flew higher still, hovering, wings spread wide as if suspended in time.

I gazed in wonder. *Flippy bird, is that you?*

The wind howled as it rattled the windows; rain pelting against the sill disguising the annoying drip. *What are you doing? It's wild out there and you'll be blown away.*

Squinting through the mist I could just make out his shape and holding my breath I waited, watched - suspended mid-air with the bird.

How can you do that? Stay strong against such force.

His wings quivered as the wind demanded he go another way; to bend to its power and give in. I could feel his struggle as he held determined, his strength measured as the seconds passed. He stayed, I stayed - the wind increased and still he held.

And then in a flash he was gone, plunging below my line of sight.

'Wow, that was amazing,' I laughed, 'what a bird you are.'

Instead of taking a leisurely bath, you somersault and flip the world upside down. You sing a song unknown to the average currawong and when the forces of nature stack against you – you hold your ground.

Are you testing yourself? Testing your strength?

Challenging a far greater power?

Who can know the mind of a bird?, I wondered.

One thing is certain: you made a choice. You decided you'd stand firm and then decided when you'd let go.

'What a special bird you are,' I whispered.

It was at that moment the thought came to me.

It was clear, it was as clear as the bird I had seen before my eyes. I had to make a change. I thought for a moment, I knew it would not be easy.

My mind worked hard around the idea that was starting to form. I slowly sat up. This was tricky. I had never focused totally on myself before. I'd have to be careful with energy. I'd have to pace myself each day. What about Steve?

I knew he would embrace the idea so I looked at it from

THE PLAN

all angles. What if I couldn't cope? Would it be adding even more pressure on us both? Lockdown was already stressful.

Stress plus more stress ... didn't add up well.

It would be hard, a lot of extra pressure, pressure I didn't need, and added expectation from Steve. I had no idea what to expect and needed to keep it simple. I'd try it alone, and if things went pear shaped ... I'd fess up.

It was at that point, I started to devise a plan to get off the opioids.

I had been taking opioids to manage chronic pain for six years. I had no idea what life would mean without them. I knew I might never get another opportunity to find out. Never before had there been so much time at my disposal. Never before had I had a break from work or from taking care of others.

Never before had I considered myself worthy.

Never before had I set such a goal.

Never before had I been so afraid.

What if the pain went out of control?

What if I couldn't cope?

What if I was back where I started?

What if ... I failed.

I considered it all, searched deep inside and acknowledged my fear. It was real – it didn't back down. I now knew what it was like to reach deep inside and take a look. I had learnt that being completely honest with myself, without judgement, could reveal truth. I also knew that truth could bring about change, and change for the better.

It wasn't easy looking inside this way, but I now understood that whatever was lurking there would not consume me. I could simply take a look, observe and then decide what I needed to do when ready – there was no longer expectation.

At last! Eureka!

I then realised I would have to do everything in my power to set it up to work. I would give it my best shot ... and that was all I could do, that was all that was required.

Lockdown now meant something else entirely.

Possibility.

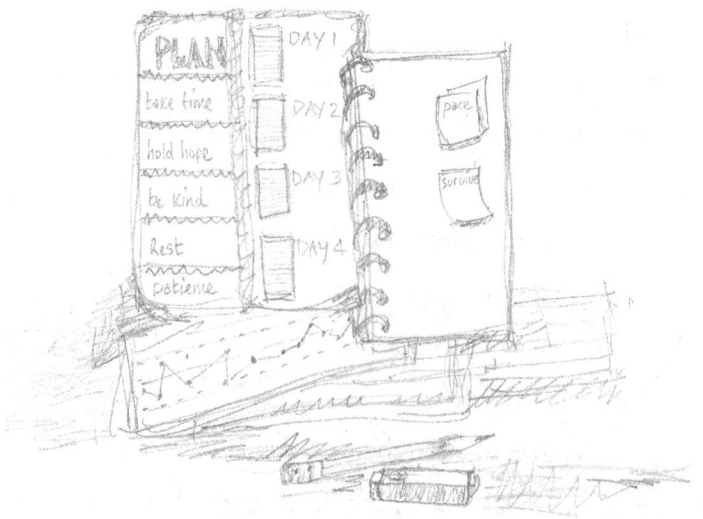

CHAPTER 31

The Plan

There were lists. I was good with lists. I loved them. I would start with identifying detail and then reduce it to point form. Nothing was spared my scrutiny. The plan was set and I was now officially my own project. Getting off the drugs was the goal, staying sane, married and alive were the priorities.

The only time I had ventured to ask a health professional the best approach to do this, I was met with mild irritation. 'May I say … you should be grateful that you are able to function on such a low dose … best not to consider that as an option … at this stage.' That was a long time ago. It's easy to get lost in the cracks.

I was only too aware that the drugs had saved me. They were prescribed at a time when I was swimming in pain and was about to drown. I was grateful. I remembered the time spent in hospital and shivered. That was the past, a place I never wanted to revisit, even though it sometimes haunted my dreams.

I contacted my GP to discuss the plan. It was agreed.

It was the great unknown and I had no idea how my body would react. Would the pain be uncontrollable? Would I be able to cope? How long would it take? Were the drugs hiding something else? Would it be too much on Steve? There were so many questions, which kept going around and round in my head, looping and weaving until I felt tied up in knots. I had to put a stop to them or they would pull me down. Another piece of clean paper was the answer and so I focused intently.

What would I do if things did get out of control pain-wise? I needed a back-up team, a team I could trust. There were techniques that had worked in the past, so I wrote them down, prioritising their effectiveness.

Ice, rest, meditation, focus, music, breathing, gentle stretches, pictures of beautiful places I loved, words of reassurance and confirmation. Some other supportive medications, such as Panadol, anti-inflammatories, creams and rubs would also be support crew.

An idea without a plan is just a wish.

THE PLAN

"Sports periodization is the systematic planning of athletic or physical training. It involves progressive cycling of various aspects of training in a specific period. The aim is to reach the best possible performance at the exact time required."

– Based on Hans Selye's General Adaption Syndrome, 1936

Starting at the end result I worked backwards, setting a timeline over the six-week period of lockdown. I loved charts almost as much as lists, and once colour coded it started to look like something I wanted to do.

Steve was aware I was up to something. I'd been very focused and a little elusive, so decided to tell him, 'I am going to focus on my own health over the next six weeks, and put a few thoughts about this down on paper.' Something must have made sense because he seemed satisfied, and was officially off my case.

It was then I realised I'd forgotten something crucial. I had better prepare some meals ahead of time, just in case I was in no fit state to function at that level, so I cooked.

This was no chore, because I knew why it was needed and cooking was always such a joy. I was doing everything I could think of ... that was in my power ... to control any possible obstacle. The freezer was full. Steve was buoyant with the selection on offer. The stage was set.

Week one commenced. I was by no means a fool and knew I would need to tread carefully and safely.

I would decrease slowly.

Skipping a dose every second day seemed the sensible option and by the end of the week I noticed that the pain was a little more present but felt I could manage it. It was saying … 'Hello'.

So far … so good … the freezer remained full.

Week two commenced. The dose was extended by a day.

Something had shifted.

Restless sleep. I tossed and turned. I walked the apartment late into the night, roaming each room, trying to think of nothing in particular, trying not to wake Steve.

I knew that too many more sleepless nights would work against me, I'd be tired, strung out, and my emotions would then start to take over proceedings. I could easily become a mess.

I had to make a tough call. I would go back to the first-week scenario and skip every other day. I reminded myself I would have to work with it gently, be patient and work with yourself … gently. There's time – respect that and give time – the space it needs.

Things settled and sleep was restored.

Time seemed to hold a different rhythm.

I was focused, but was strangely in a daze.

THE PLAN

Week three commenced. The days blurred and halfway into the third week, I decided to try extending the extra day again. It threw out the schedule a little, but I felt it was time.

I wrote everything down to track what was happening, and kept a record of my body's reactions. I was finding it hard to focus.

At the end of that week I was feeling aches and pains elsewhere in my body, deep, deep, deep in my bones. I started my gentle releases and added a few more hot showers. I didn't feel right. My head ached and the Panadol was not doing its job. Day three of this scenario brought nose bleeds, three in one day. Should I back off again? I could usually trust my instinct, but I was not feeling good.

There were hot flushes and unexpected hits of anxiety.

The nausea caught Steve's attention.

He was worried. 'What on *earth* is happening here? You look like death warmed up … have you caught something?'

I fessed up.

Steve knew me very well and he was more aware of the situation than I gave credit.

While I was focusing on myself, attempting to relax and go with the flow, he was observing an entirely different scenario.

He watched the shaky hands take the teacup from him in the morning, all the while trying to steady the cup and not spill a drop. He listened to the mutterings while I was preparing dinner. He saw me shift and change position, time and again, unable to stand still in one spot. He felt the shifts in energy. He'd notice me frantically cleaning one day, and unable to get out of bed the next. He knew I wasn't listening to him.

I may have looked the same, but my eyes said something completely different.

Steve held me close as I dissolved into tears.

'Oh Poss you are such a brave girl … but you don't need to be the Lone Ranger on this one … let's work together on this and then it's two against one … what do you say?'

I could say nothing, my mind was a scramble. My head was pounding and I wasn't exactly sure which of the back-up team was needed. I stayed in his arms and sobbed.

This was the best support any girl could hope for and at exactly the right time. My body relaxed with the breath and using my sleeve to mop up my face, I attempted a weak smile and for the first time in weeks looked into Steve's eyes.

How foolish I'd been to underestimate the power of love.

Had I learnt nothing?

In the spirit of reconciliation, Steve made us a very large cafe latte. There were plenty of Anzac biscuits due to the recent baking frenzy, and so we agreed to indulge with two. As Steve chomped into his third he declared, 'This is cause for celebration, after all … and we both need stamina to see it through.'

THE PLAN

The news was banned. There was nothing in it that helped our personal stress, so Steve announced, 'I'll be the filter on how things are progressing, and will keep you informed when it's necessary.'

I stayed in bed. It was raining heavily and there was nothing I desperately needed to do. I dozed and tossed amid strange dreams.

The last few days or nights were a muddle.

I was in a huge house full of stairs. There were rooms on different levels, with stairs leading to another room, another room, another room. Some of them spiralled upwards and others went straight to another level.

And then I saw my mother, seated on a chair, reading a book. She looked up and smiled. I asked her what she was doing there? She said, this is where she lived.

I asked her was she happy there? She said she was, but she would appreciate a glass of water.

I was so pleased to see my mother. So pleased to see her happy. I turned to go down the stairs to look for some water, and found I was somewhere else entirely. I didn't know the way back. I didn't know where I was.

And woke with a start.

My heart was pounding out of my chest and in a sweat, I reached for the glass of water with shaking hands. 'Oh my goodness, that was ... interesting.'

The tears were flowing uncontrollably. I wiped and wiped. There was no sound, no words, there was nothing other than tears. I sniffed my way through a box of tissues and then lay back in bed exhausted.

The next thing I knew, Steve was standing next to the bed. It was dark. 'Are you ok in there?'

I turned slowly and tried to focus. 'What time is it?'

'After 8 pm and you ... Poss ... must have something to eat.'

I felt weak and drained. I slowly lifted myself onto my elbows and nodded.

Week four commenced. Time dragged. I was there and then I wasn't. It was as if someone else had taken over my body and I had no comprehension of who, or where I was.

Days morphed into more days. There were meals, sometimes there were none because of the nausea. Sometimes I found myself staring into the courtyard, waiting ... waiting for God knows what.

Other times I tried reading the same line of my book over and over again. I saw the light reflecting on the birdbath. I saw it - nothing more than that. Time waited with me.

Steve was the only constant. He supported, he encouraged, he placed the soup in front of me.

He smiled when I missed half the conversation and answered a previous question.

THE PLAN

He was doing the best he could. I was mostly somewhere else, an unknown place which felt like an empty void.

'Sorry, did you say something?' I asked, as Steve walked down the stairs towards me.

'I've been saying something for the last five minutes – have you heard nothing of the conversation?'

I looked up. I was preparing dinner and was miles away. Shaking his head, he gave up.

'What was it?' I stopped chopping veggies so I could concentrate on him.

'It doesn't matter now, only that lockdown looks to extend and we'll be stuck in the bunker for a while longer.'

'Oh? Do you know how long?'

'Could be weeks,' he shrugged, 'no one really knows.'

I nodded, taking in his words. Thinking was an effort and took all my concentration. Pain levels were constantly present, but I was managing with rest, Panadol and icepacks.

There was no concept of myself. I had become very small.

I didn't know what the date was, but I did know that the dose was every four days and the prepared charts were working.

The blur of lockdown mixed with the blur in my mind.

I could note down each day and not have to strain to remember what had just happened. I looked back through the list and realised that I was more than halfway through.

Where did that go?

The frozen meals I had carefully prepared were easy for Steve to maintain. I could do this and I smiled. It had been a long time since I had felt anything so I drew a smiley face on the day and coloured it in for good measure.

I took a shower and rummaged through my wardrobe. Steve was doing some computer work in the second bedroom.

I hadn't been anywhere near this room I realised, so gently knocked on the door. He said something.

I opened the door and waited at the entry. Still seated, he slowly turned around. Nothing could prepare me for the look on his face.

He was staring wide eyed … staring … mouth open … staring.

'Well … I don't know who you are, but it sure is nice to meet you … did you just walk in off the street or something? Wait 'til my wife gets wind of this.'

Orecchiette with Broccoli

Ingredients:

400 g orecchiette

2 garlic cloves (finely chopped)

1 pinch dried chilli flakes

1 brown onion (finely chopped)

½ teaspoon honey

2 large broccoli heads (cut into bite size florets)

2 cups chicken stock (heated)

1 tablespoon roasted pine nuts

Zest and juice of 1 lemon

Splash of Worcestershire sauce and tomato sauce

Parmesan cheese

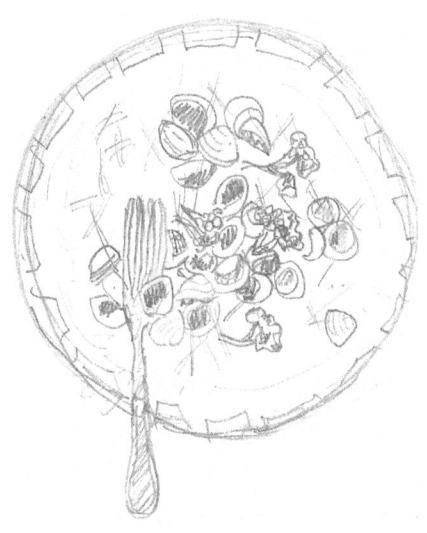

Method:

In a medium size saucepan, bring chicken stock to the boil.

Prepare washed broccoli into bite size florets.

In a non-stick frying pan with a little olive oil, cook onion, garlic, chilli flakes and honey, until translucent.

Add the dried orecchiette, and stir until warm and coated with the flavours.

Gradually add the hot chicken stock, as you would for risotto, allowing the pasta to absorb the stock before adding more.

Add both sauces, lemon juice and zest.

Continue to add the stock until half cooked.

Add the broccoli over the top and place a lid to steam.

Keep checking the liquid and adding if necessary.

When the broccoli is bright green and still crunchy, add the pine nuts and mix.

Serve:

Serve with a drizzle of olive oil, parmesan cheese and crusty bread.

THE PLAN

CHAPTER 32

The Best Is Yet To Come

"Give me your world, and I'll give you heaven. Love will set us free, as long as we believe, the best is yet to come"
- Song written by Cynthia Biggs & Dexter Wansel
- Recorded by Patti Labelle & Grover Washington, 1982

I lay on the stretch mat. We had just been for a short walk around the block and it was my turn to go through my gentle releases, on the floor.

Week five commenced. Steve and I had decided that a small walk combining stretches each day was a good idea. The walk was determined by the weather and Steve's work routine.

It's something we could easily manage and brought a sense of rhythm and focus to the day.

I was now looking forward to seeing our neighbourhood, instead of hiding from it. Gradually we increased how far we walked, until it became easier and I felt stronger.

Gently, I walked. Slowly, I managed.

Looking to the sky and beyond, I allowed myself to breathe.

To stop if I needed to, to speed up, if I was able.

To take in the trees, to feel the cold air on my face.

Allowing time … allowing space.

Allowing time and space … to heal.

Steve was thinking of dinner. We had just finished the leftover capsicum and lentil soup for lunch, and already he was checking out the fridge.

I smiled to myself, some things were very predictable and thank goodness for that.

'Would you like me to cook tonight's dinner? I could … I'm a good cook you know!'

I moved onto my back and started the glute stretches. Oh yes, I knew he could cook, it was more the creative mess that was associated with the cook up, that didn't really inspire me. 'Yes … that would be lovely thank you … do we have any broccoli? Your broccoli orecchiette is very good.'

The rain was relentless. There had been no walks for two days and we were both missing our routine. We still stretched, but going outside lifted our spirits and we realised just how important it had become.

Lockdown meant we were all stuck in a weird holding pattern, where meals, exercise, social interaction and home schooling blurred together under the same roof. Some friends coped by designating certain days for certain things. Mondays meant cooking vegetarian, Tuesdays for washing, Wednesdays cleaning, Thursdays a roast of some description, Friday pasta, Saturday football and Sunday take-away food … a day off cooking, a break from the norm.

Finding some kind of normal was essential or we would all struggle to remain sane. Creating a sense of structure meant our lives weren't really out of our control.

Outdoor neighbouring brick walls became tennis ball targets and someone we knew, determined to increase their golf handicap in lockdown, installed a net to catch the hundreds of golf balls flying in all directions. We didn't have outdoor space to play in our apartment but we enjoyed watching our friends Zoom their surroundings.

Marian often sent me a video of their farm.

She understood the restrictions of our four walls, and seeing the early morning mist rise from the dam, the chickens fighting to roost in a pot plant or the children chasing each other around the yard, cheered us up. It was real. It was life.

We could see the horizon, the clouds, the grass and trees moving in the breeze, and as they fired up the BBQ we could almost smell the breakfast cooking, laughing as we pretended to bite a sausage offered to the screen. It was being involved. Being connected. Being somewhere else.

Having to stay indoors so long really highlighted the importance of home and even though apartment living didn't offer the flexibilities that a house and yard can give, it was our safe haven and we were grateful.

I was hanging up the second load of washing, and poor Steve was now surrounded. It was the warmest place in the apartment and clothes were shuffled around the room and Steve, on their wire racks, manoeuvred according to thickness, length and need.

The sheets and towels were next and I was just about to strip the bed, when I heard the call.

'Dwoh, dwoh, dwoh.'

I looked up in a flash ... waited ... and there it was again.

'Dwoh, dwoh, dwoh.'

Moving to the bedroom window, I opened the blinds and looked out. It was nearing dusk, and even though the clouds were grey, they held a touch of pink as the sun slipped behind the buildings in front of me.

When had I last heard that call? I honestly couldn't remember. In fact, I couldn't recall much of the last five weeks.

Scanning the trees beyond, I was looking for a sign.

Just as I was about to turn away, I heard the reply.

'Dweh, dweh, dweh.'

Then I saw them. In fact, it was only one to begin.

It flew directly across the sky and out of sight.

I smiled and whispered, 'Flippy bird, how wonderful.' 'Dweh, dweh, dweh … dweh, dweh, dweh' following immediately after.

The sense of urgency in that call suggested it was quite irritated or excited, or something. The expectation that it was to follow along behind its mate and keep followingwas wearing thin. 'Dweh, dweh, dweh … dweh, dweh, dweh …'

I watched the colour fade away in the clouds. I observed the light slowly diffuse. I stayed until the shadows deepened and the reflections became dark silhouettes.

Night had fallen. It was dark and it was beautiful. For the first time in weeks I appreciated my world – the simple beauty of it.

I realised something important. I'd been living in lockdown for years. Pain had demanded it. Time passed by around it.

Thinking clearly made me smile. I rubbed my back to reduce the ache, reassuring myself it would pass.

I could never bring myself to thank the virus for lockdown, but as I contemplated the darkness, I realised it had given back my life.

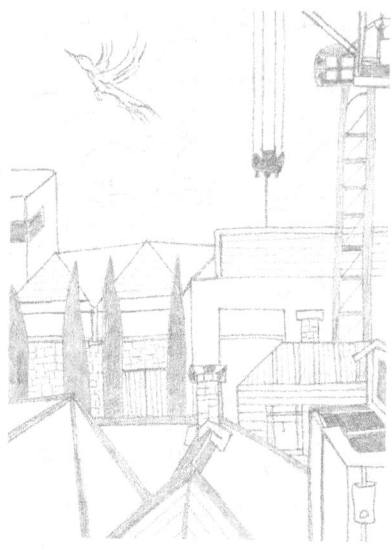

A few lights flickered on in the apartments opposite and I could see the shadow of a person walk to a window and look out. We were doing the same, both looking out. Different lives. Different struggles. Looking out beyond ourselves.

In that precious moment I realised I was coming back to life and I knew, with a simple bird call ... that there was hope.

"Winter, spring, summer or fall, all you have to do is call, and I'll be there, yes I will ... you've got a friend"
– *James Taylor & Carole King, 1971*

I checked my phone. I had turned it off. I had wanted to relax from the pressure of the world and what I didn't expect were the number of messages waiting for me.

THE BEST IS YET TO COME

Clients were concerned. I hadn't responded to their messages, and they were worried about me. I made a list and responded.

They were not aware of my personal goal over this period, and so I reassured them that I was ok, needing time to focus on my own health. They were so kind, and I felt privileged to call many of them friends.

The last message stopped me in my tracks. Marian had left three messages; the last one brought tears to my eyes.

After giving myself a moment to regroup, I rang her. She would be busy with home schooling, so I listened to her voicemail message bank and left a reply. I made a cup of tea and thought how fortunate I was to have Marian in my life.

How I had come to deserve such a friend, I would never know but like many chance meetings, we were thrown together unexpectedly, and seemed to click easily into friendship.

We had both attended a very average life coaching course years before. I had completed my personal training studies and wanted to broaden my skills by becoming a life coach.

We had bonded after the first week, and gradually shared our thoughts about life, and the inconsistencies of the course material. I had met a fellow organiser and list maker, and felt that this in itself was money well spent on the course.

The owner of the coaching firm must have been aware there

was something different about us because, to our amusement, we were invited to a meeting to discuss the possibility of becoming directors of the company.

Sitting in a café, we listened and nodded, sipped our coffee, and thanked them for the kind offer. Without having a discussion, we had both made the same 'no thanks' reply. Escaping to another café, we debriefed and realised that we were very much alike.

'Well ... that was interesting ... did you get a strange vibe during that meeting? I couldn't get away quickly enough, something just didn't feel right.'

And so it began, our lives intertwined. I came out of retirement to sing at Marian's wedding. No one knew it at the time, but the song was the prediction of their future lives together. Marriage brought with it a shift to the country to manage the family farm and also the best possible gift that life could give.

"Will you stay with me, will you be my love, among the fields of barley?"
— *Sting, 1993, 'Fields of Gold'*

I was now a proud godmother. Grace was the delightful bundle of joy that accompanied us shopping, walking around the streets of Carlton, and visiting every playground in the vicinity.

BRING ON SPRING

After a number of years, Dean arrived and the little family blossomed amid the fields of barley.

I was amazed how the city dwellers had adapted to country living. Admittedly, Mark had grown up on this farm; he'd experienced the rigours of raising sheep and cattle and the demands farm life took on family. Marian also understood farming. Her family had a stone fruit orchard in the Shepparton district and many school holidays were spent in packing sheds frantically getting the fruit harvest to market.

This couple were a horticultural match made in heaven. Educated, smart and capable of mixing with a broad range of people, they quickly became involved in the community. We soon heard about events they supported, helping raise money for the SES, local fire services and schools the children attended.

Many years ago we'd visited Mark and Marian's farm and stayed in the old original farmhouse. I remember hugging five-year-old Grace as we sat on the front steps looking out across the surrounding fields. Playing 'I-spy' was easy because she was observant and knew the farm well. We quickly moved on from spying the dam, ducks, the cattle and trees and focused on a stone, a gate and a dragonfly.

Once Grace had exhausted the game she took me on a tour of the place: where the chickens lived, the hammock strung up on the veranda and the ancient woolshed where the sheep were sheared. As soon as we walked in we could smell the musty scent of wool. Light filtered through the old wooden slats sending dust particles dancing through the air.

It was beautiful and Grace beamed with pride as she told me how the sheep shivered when their woolly coats fell to the floor. The wooden barn felt like it might blow away in a strong wind, unlike the main residence, whose solid stone walls and high ceilings gave the impression it would outlive us all.

The original landholding dated to the 1800s and the homestead itself had history; it was a survivor.

Mark's parents purchased the property in the 1970s and transformed the place. They were still involved in the farm when we visited and lived in the local village, transitioning to retirement … they were gradually letting go of their life's work.

It's not easy letting go. Especially when a lifetime of blood, sweat and tears have been given to the land, given to every fence post, every nail in every shed, every paddock and every piece of machinery.

It's also not easy to be patient. Mark and Marian were in the process of purchasing the farm and this transition was taking time.

I have to admit, some of the best conversations I've had in my life have been shared with Marian.

I can't say we've solved many issues, but once we've exhausted ourselves covering all aspects of a subject, there's a sense we might be a little wiser, even more aware than when we started.

Honesty can open doors you didn't know were shut. It can reveal the truth within ourselves and provide answers to questions which have not been asked. Patience is a topic we often discussed and after years of debate, we've decided it's a wise woman who can recognise her own impatience and then with good humour, promptly file it away under control freak.

'Hello friends Mark and I have been talking … and we think it would be wonderful … if you both would like to consider … after lockdown … or before the next one … to come and live with us for a while. The change would do you good … country air … and we miss you.'

My heart could not be contained. This was what Marian was like. She had the ability to say or do exactly the right thing … at exactly the right moment. Both Steve and I loved this family, and we felt part of them somehow.

We were touched beyond measure and would treasure this offer for the rest of our lives.

A CURRAWONG SOMERSAULT

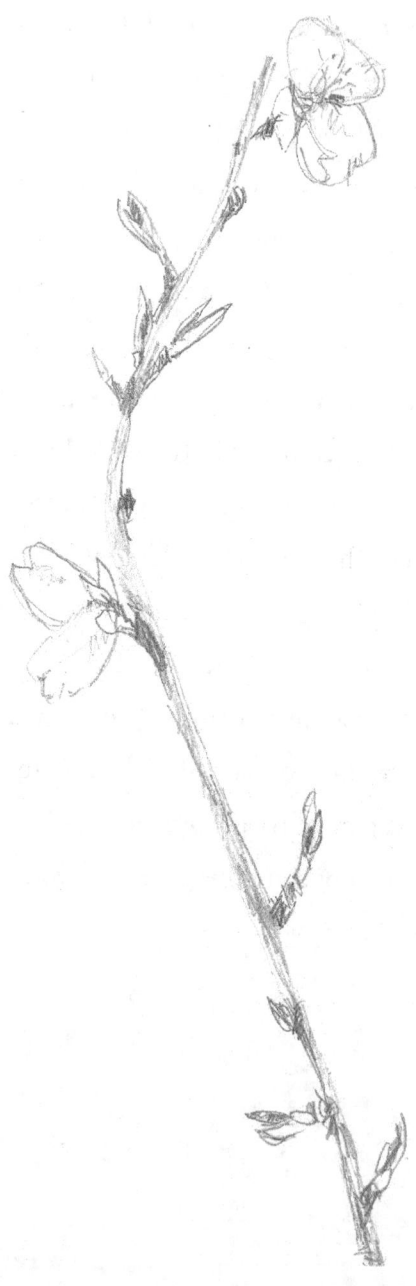

CHAPTER 33

Bring on Spring

All the leaves had gone. The trees were bare but already little buds could be seen, as they waited expectantly for the next season's arrival. Spring always brought a sense of hope.

I love Spring. The fresh new growth, vibrant colours, the blossoms with their fragrant smells, but most of all, I love the excited behaviour of all the birdlife that surround us.

There are more baths at this time, and often a queue, with little birds sitting high in the trees, waiting until the larger ones have dried off.

It is wonderful. I would need to be patient, and wait with the buds.

I looked to the sky. There was grey cloud. I couldn't imagine what it would be like to be in a country that didn't have definite seasons. Living with constant grey would be very challenging, with or without COVID.

At least I knew, without a doubt, that Spring would bring with it a welcome change. I wondered about the future. It was hard to look ahead and see a vision of it. It was blurry.

I wondered whether my business would ever recover.

I wondered, almost … not daring to wonder.

Would the *World's Most Livable City* survive?

Looking up I saw a blonde head stride past the kitchen window. I hadn't seen Louis for a while, and so made my way to the front door, catching him wee on the wall near our front door. 'Oh no! Sorry! Louis you naughty boy … he clearly couldn't wait to get outside … so sorry!' I smiled and bent down to give the excited dog an energetic rub. 'Oh he's fine a dog's gotta do what a dog's gotta do … eh Louis? Oh you are such a handsome boy … do you realise that?' Of course he did, and jumped into my arms.

The virus numbers were rising and I was beginning to wonder whether COVID Stage 4 restrictions would soon be introduced. So far, I hadn't heard of anyone I knew who had contracted the virus but it was certainly present.

Victoria now had a total of 4,750 cases and 29 deaths. New cases were increasing daily, each succeeding the last record.

BRING ON SPRING

Today was 317 cases and I was beginning to feel uneasy. Was it closing in?

Megan rang and she sounded slightly agitated. She had purchased masks and had done her shopping, stocking up in case there were further outbreaks in her area. So far things were clear.

Her GP was working alone, because everyone else in the clinic had been traced to the virus. One patient was the carrier and the whole clinic shut down because of that. Megan was spooked and as I listened, I couldn't help but feel the same.

This was real.

This was getting closer. This didn't feel very good.

We chatted about everything else we could possibly think of that wasn't looming front and centre in our minds: any distraction from reality.

Thank goodness for football. We discussed the coaching strategies of many teams, until I couldn't help bringing up Geelong's recent win.

All the AFL teams had been relocated to other territories so they could stay safe, and continue playing the game. Round 7 was Geelong vs Collingwood, so I was feeling optimistic after my team's last impressive win against the Gold Coast Suns.

It was a wonderful game. The total Geelong team were present and accounted for and when that happens, they are a force to be reckoned with.

Captain Joel Selwood clocked his 300th game and Gary Ablett Junior played his 350th. It was momentous. Megan agreed, I had every right to feel proud. She was waiting for the Saints to win a game, her fingers cramping after being crossed for so long.

Megan hung up.

I stood for a while … silent.

'Stay safe my dear friend … stay very safe.'

Steve had made our second cafe latte. It was better than the first, as he honed his skill in lockdown.

He had ground another bag of beans, and the smell filled the lower ground floor apartment. 'Gosh that smells amazing. I wonder can you ingest caffeine this way? It's so strong … mmm … we just need to add milk somehow.'

I wished I hadn't spoken. Thankfully Steve had missed half the conversation, with the noise of the steamer gurgling in the background.

Sometimes he could be a tad unpredictable, so I changed the subject.

'Should we go to the market early tomorrow morning? What do you think? It feels so much safer at that hour … some people simply don't get distancing … let's buy some salmon and … do a pappardelle … would you like that?'

I knew that I never needed to ask Steve any of these questions; he would love to go to the market … the earlier the better ... and salmon pappardelle, with capers, anchovies, red onion, garlic and dill was one of his all-time favourites.

Yes. Yes. And Yes.

He went upstairs, to complete any urgent business, which he effectively did online.

I contemplated my day. It looked much the same as yesterday, except for the waft of coffee still in the air. Sighing, I realised how simple our lives had become. Steve spent most of his time in the office upstairs managing his business remotely, on his computer and phone. I was either downstairs, or in bed, depending on how my pain was. Every day blurred into the next until a week blended into many, as the seasons changed.

We added layers of clothing to soften Winter's evening chill; track pants and windcheaters, woolly socks and scarves meant hibernation, warmth, and a safe place to be. And then, just as you'd rearranged your wardrobe, warmer weather required tops and T-shirts which started the reshuffle all over again.

Standing by myself, I looked out to the courtyard. It was too early to expect any birds to visit the bath and it would be ridiculous to wait here until the afternoon parade began. There was a lull in the neighbouring construction site. The noise of machinery, which surrounded and took over our small courtyard, had subsided, making this silence seem deafening. I stood, waiting for the world to shift around me to reconfigure and wipe the dreadful coronavirus from our lives.

How many times had I stood like this? How many times had I negotiated with myself? How to remain sane in lockdown ...

No doubt there'll be years of study associated with the long-term mental health effects of being closed in. Medical experts will be tracking the psychological changes to children and adults in years to come, evaluating the effects COVID-19 restrictions have brought to our lives.

How long would we be living like this?

Not knowing was the killer.

No one could accurately predict the impact of COVID-19 and future ramifications of the global pandemic for Australia.

I could still smell coffee. Was it too early to start dinner?

Of course it was and anyway, I'd made double serves of pasta the day before so I could avoid the routine dinner plan. Steve was lucky. He was good at compartmentalising. He could blissfully troll through countless hours online ... until the smell of food made him hungry. I sometimes wished I had a brain that could easily stay entertained for hours on end.

I was more of a search and find and then move on type of person ... getting side-tracked by new information wasn't something I slipped into easily.

Happiness for me was a project with a definite focus … guided by a process which I followed until the final outcome. It had been a difficult experience making my recovery into a project. I found it challenging focusing on myself, recognising my weakness and working through my fears.

Achieving my goal is one of the hardest things I have ever done and getting off opioids and working with the unpredictability of withdrawal has challenged me to the core. My physical and mental struggle is still a work in progress … and I felt tired.

Tired of myself.

Tired of lockdown.

Tired of being tired.

I went to the kitchen window and looked out.

How many times had I done this?

This year had become the year of windows, so much looking out. A stranger walked past. I stood still. The same woman walked past again, this time her arms were full of boxes. I went to the front door, she had gone. Looking down made me smile. 'Oh hello … and who do we have here?'

Sitting on the front mat was a shaggy white dog, with floppy ears and an overbite only a mother could be proud of. 'Oh hi,' said the owner, 'this is Nelly and she's very sociable … so sorry she's disturbed you … we've just moved in.'

I laughed, tousling the shaggy head, 'Oh don't worry, I'm sure we'll meet again very soon … welcome to our 'hood.'

I stood alone in the doorway, leant forward to catch a glimpse of sky. Waiting. The sky was bright and the breeze hinted that someone nearby was cooking with chilli. Looking down at the empty doormat, I smiled. Yes … life can be like that, it can be unpredictable and throw the unexpected your way.

We never know what's around the corner. Our well-made plans can be turned upside down in an instant. We may think we will never survive when shock or disaster strikes, but survive we do. Back injury and chronic pain brought me to my knees but it also taught me how to stand tall and gradually draw strength and happiness from the simplest of things.

Love of our beautiful world and the people around us can offer healing and a better understanding of ourselves. The sun rises and sets, bringing a new day and the idea that anything is possible.

Tough times? Perhaps … but then, you never know what might turn up on your front step. And if you're lucky it just might have four legs and a wagging tail.

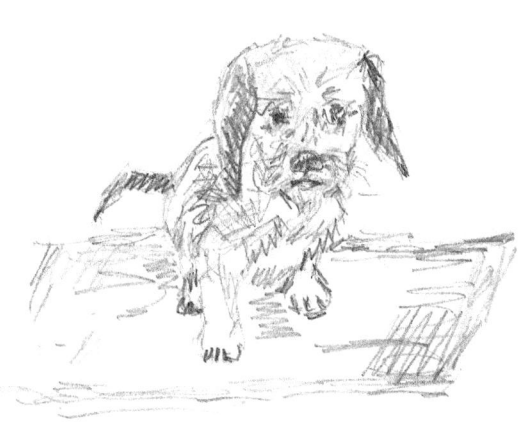

Salmon Pappardelle with Red Onion and Dill

Ingredients:
Pappardelle pasta
1 red onion (finely chopped)
2 garlic cloves (finely chopped)
2 teaspoons capers
1 large piece salmon (finely sliced, no skin)
1 pinch chilli flakes
½ teaspoon honey
1 tablespoon thickened cream or crème fraiche
3-4 anchovies (chopped)
½ bunch dill (coarsely chopped)
1 tablespoon pan roasted pine nuts
Zest of 1 lemon

Method:

In a fry pan, gently cook onion, garlic, anchovies and chilli flakes in a little olive oil, until translucent.

Add the honey, capers and reduce heat to caramelise.

In a large saucepan, bring water to the boil.

In the meantime, slice the salmon ready and finish other prep.

Cook pasta until just 'al dente'.

Drain liquid into a bowl and reserve.

Transfer pasta into the pan, adding the dill, pine nuts, and salmon.

Gently toss until salmon is nearly cooked.

Add lemon zest and lastly the cream.

Add some of the reserved liquid to loosen the pasta.

Season to taste.

Serve:
Serve with fresh baguette and your best red wine.

About the Author

Heather Walker is a first-time author who has drawn on her personal experience to deliver a message of hope and encouragement to anyone who is experiencing challenge.

She has been working in her personal training business in Melbourne Victoria for 20 years and is a qualified Train the Trainer, life coach and stretch therapist, specialising in rehabilitation, older adults and pregnancy.

Over the last few years she has developed a unique observation-based method of working with clients, in response to a back injury which left her physically living with the restrictions of chronic pain.

Prior to this she enjoyed a professional singing career spanning 20 years, which involved performing around Australia and TV appearances, and co-wrote and performed the show *I'll Take Manhattan*, a tribute to the Manhattan Transfer, in venues around Melbourne.

She grew up in regional country Victoria, moving to Adelaide for 10 years and then Melbourne to further her musical studies and career. While living in Adelaide she taught pianoforte, singing, performed professionally and provided part-time assistance with the United Marion Care program for the underprivileged.

She proudly calls Melbourne home – *The World's Most Livable City* – and resides there with her husband.

Quotes, References & Songs

		Page
1.	"When something doesn't work one way, you have to find another." – Nanna Wilson	88
2.	"All good things must come to an end." – Geoffrey Chaucer, poet, 1380s, *Troilus and Criseyde*	94
3.	"From little things big things grow." – Paul Kelly, songwriter, 1993	95
4.	"Survival mode is a short-term, fear based mode of thinking that you enter when your flight-or-fight response is triggered." – Heather Walker	184
5.	'Softly, softly how does it grow? Gently, gently where butterflies land, opening, closing, finding a way, slowly reveal the depths of things you can't say.' – Heather Walker	187
6.	"We don't need to find a set up where someone wins and someone loses." – Jimmy Bonduc, 1992, 'Let Me Be the One'	206
7.	"A sense of humour is the best indicator that you will recover, sustain that and you have hope." – Andrew Solomon, 2000, from *The Noonday Demon – An Atlas of Depression*	248
8.	"Jesu Joy of Man's Desiring." – J. S. Bach, 1716, Cantata 147	252
9.	"Clowns to the left of me, jokers to the right, here I am, stuck in the middle with you." – Steelers Wheel, 1972 (Gerry Rafferty & Joe Egan)	287

10. "In Freudian psychology and psychoanalysis, the reality principal, is the ability of the mind to assess the reality of the external world, and to act upon it accordingly, as opposed to acting on the pleasure principal."
    – Sigmund Freud, 1896, Reality Principal 306

11. Human nature – "The natural ways of behaving that most people share"
    – Cambridge University Dictionary 316

12. "Desperate times call for desperate measures."
    – Hippocrates, 1500 BC 337

13. "Sports periodization – is the systematic planning of athletic or physical training. It involves progressive cycling of various aspects of training in a specific period. The aim is to reach the best performance at the exact time required."
    – Based on Hans Selye's General Adaption Syndrome, 1936 343

14. "The best is yet to come ... Give me your world ... love will set us free ... as long as we believe the best is yet to come."
    – Song written by Cynthia Biggs & Dexter Wansel, 1982 353

15. "Winter, spring, summer, or fall, all you have to do is call, and I'll be there, yes I will ... you've got a friend."
    – James Taylor & Carole King, 1971 358

16. "Will you stay with me, will you be my love, among the fields of barley."
    – Sting, 1993, 'Fields of Gold' 360

Acknowledgements

With thanks to my proof-reader, Adam. A special thank you to Chris for her invaluable help and support. To Margaret for her input and to Jill for suggesting I write a book.

www.ingramcontent.com/pod-product-compliance
Lightning Source LLC
Chambersburg PA
CBHW050259010526
44107CB00055B/2089